A Nine-Stage Roadmap to **Recover Energy,**
Reverse Chronic Illness, *and Claim the Potential of a*
Vibrant New You

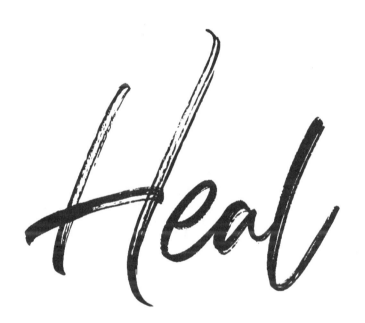

Karyn Shanks MD

Fatigue is Not Your Destiny

Cover design and graphics by Robin Deutschendorf,
Brown Wing Studio, Iowa City, IA.

Print ISBN: 978-1-7339176-0-5
E-Book ISBN: 978-1-7339176-1-2

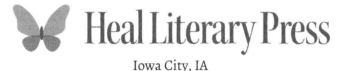

Heal Literary Press
Iowa City, IA
HealLiteraryPress.com

First Edition

The Nine Domains of Healing Roadmap

A Bird's-Eye View of Our Terrain

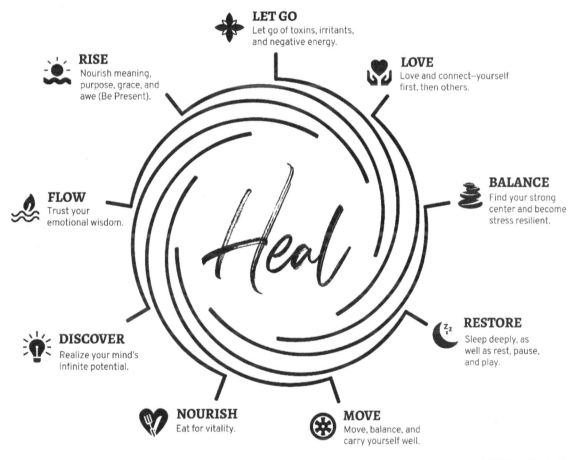

LET GO
Let go of toxins, irritants, and negative energy.

RISE
Nourish meaning, purpose, grace, and awe (Be Present).

LOVE
Love and connect—yourself first, then others.

FLOW
Trust your emotional wisdom.

BALANCE
Find your strong center and become stress resilient.

DISCOVER
Realize your mind's infinite potential.

RESTORE
Sleep deeply, as well as rest, pause, and play.

NOURISH
Eat for vitality.

MOVE
Move, balance, and carry yourself well.

Heal

For Brian: My angel.

HEAL
\hēl

Haelan (Old English), Hailjan (Proto-Germanic)
—to make whole.

Not perfect.

Not unscathed by life.

Not without scars or suffering.

But real. Fully lived. Unbroken. Holy.

A life made more beautiful and whole by braving, living, and nourishing an authentic life.

CONTENTS

MANIFESTO TO A HEALING LIFE

We Care. We Hope. We Heal.

We Care.

First, we care for ourselves with great reverence.

We believe in our higher selves and embrace our soul's vast potential through care of our *whole* selves: body, mind, and spirit.

We become strong. We become whole.

Then we care for others—our families, our communities, and our world. We reach out from our strength and wholeness to share our light with those around us. We strive to elevate others and in doing so elevate our world and ourselves.

We Hope.

We know hope is the highest expression of our potential and allows us to move forward, strengthening us in the face of all life's challenges.

We allow hope to expand us: inspiring our growth and healing, making tomorrow a better day than today.

We ignite hope with clear intention and action, and throw open the doors to the infinite possibilities of our lives.

We Heal.

We know that healing is the primary urge of nature. We claim this healing as our own.

Healing is actively striving to achieve the purpose for which we were born. While not always curing, healing elevates our souls.

We know the bones of healing are in *what we do for ourselves* and in our brave, reverent attention to what matters most: our full participation in our lives, our relationships, and our world.

We heal. And our path to healing is also the prize: our radiant presence, our truest selves, our brilliant potential, our deepest healing. Our bright presence inspires others— igniting hope, illuminating our shared path.

We take this journey together.

INTRODUCTION

"I just want to be . . . *myself* . . . again," Ruth blurted out.

She seemed surprised to hear herself say it. But there it was, the essence of her greatest loss, what chronic illness had taken from her. It was the reason why she'd *really* come to see me. Years of illness, profound fatigue, and brain fog had destroyed her sense of who she was: vibrant, active, capable—*herself.*

While she came to me thinking she wanted my help to make her less sick, what she desired more, surprising even herself, was to reclaim the person she truly was. Consciously she wanted to be cured, but her deeper longing was to be healed.

This is one of the mind-blowing insights I've learned from years of listening to my clients—whose stories are just like yours. You've been taught to ask for cures, but inside you *know* you want healing. You've been told to look for ways to lower your blood sugar, lose weight, reduce inflammation, or learn to live with chronic pain or fatigue. But you aspire to something much greater than that.

You know what's really at stake here: You want your life back. You want your energy back. You want to claim the potential that you know is yours.

Yes, watching what you eat and learning ways to adapt to stress or a chronic disability are important. But inside—even if it's buried deep—in the quiet reflective time alone in bed at two in the morning, you *know* there is more. You're certain of it. That's why you're here.

From academics, to CEOs, to Iowa farmers, all my clients end up saying some version of the same thing when I ask about their goals for healing:

"I want to be *myself* again."

"I want my daughter to know the *real* me."

"I just want the energy to enjoy my family."

"I want the energy to reach my full potential."

They can. They absolutely can. And they do.

So can you. I'm not talking about the hyped up, quick fixes of the latest energy fad. We want much more than that. What we all seek is a sustainable source of deep, robust, life-giving energy. I call this Big Energy. This is the vigor, the enthusiasm, and the vibrancy that creates and sustains all of who we are and what we're capable of. Physically, mentally, spiritually, Big Energy is our potential as people.

The book in your hands addresses the central theme of all persistent fatigue, burnout, and chronic illness: energy. Energy—Big Energy—is the most powerful indicator of our level of health and vitality, and what we all seek in our healing. In this book, I reveal the roadmap—the Nine Domains of Healing— to what creates and sustains the energy you need to claim your full potential—to heal.

WHY THIS PATH? BECAUSE WE ARE ENERGY

Energy is who we are. It's what we can do. It's what allows us to dream. At some point we've all felt "in the zone." When things happen effortlessly, when we do whatever we please, and we do it well. Whether in the kitchen, on the sports field, in the boardroom, we're in the groove. We're fully present. And it feels great. It feels right. It's where we want to be. It's life.

But for many of us, there's a dark side to that story—fatigue. We've all been there, feeling it overshadow everything. Without our energy, we're swimming in mud—moving in slow, sad motion through our days. There's no way to feel inspired, happy, or satisfied when there's no gas in the tank. Life calls and we must answer—go to work, raise the kids, do our daily chores. We get by, but without energy we have little joy, little life.

Energy underpins everything that makes us who we are: all our action and behavior, our inspiration and ideas, our passion and curiosity about the world around us, and our connection to everything in our lives. Every thought, experience, and emotion is energy. It's our creative life force. Energy is the very essence of who we are.

Energy is what we lose when we are ill or feel depleted in the face of life's complexities. When the flow of who we are and where we want to be is blocked. When the potential of our lives is stomped on. We must reclaim it. We *can* reclaim it for ourselves.

Reigniting our energy is the true focus and meaning of all our efforts to heal.

MY MOST DIFFICULT PATIENT—*ME*

I've lived this low-energy story. At the age of thirty-five, I went through what I call my "universal smackdown." This was an experience that reshaped my understanding of the nature of healing, compelled me to reckon with the life stories that got in my way, and set me on a new path of how to heal and reclaim my own Big Energy.

After the weight of thirty-five years of unremitting stress, inadequate nutrition for my unique (but basically "normal") physiology, grueling medical training, two pregnancies, and carrying the weight of my family's wellbeing (and of my patients, and of the whole dang world!) on my shoulders, I crashed and burned. Yes, I still got up every day and did what I needed to. But I was completely overwhelmed, exhausted, and had lost all resilience. My body shut me down and shut me up. My Big Energy was hijacked.

Overwhelmed and exhausted, I was unable to enjoy my rich life of a loving family and the deeply meaningful work I had created. I searched for answers. I prayed for an abnormal thyroid test so that I could solve all of my problems with one simple pill, but my labs were always normal. No one could find anything wrong with me, and I was encouraged to brush off how I felt. I mean, fatigue is "normal" for a mom with two kids and a job. And migraine headaches are pretty common, right?

But I was fortunate. Through a series of serendipitous events I discovered what I needed. More than a new way to look at things, I discovered a roadmap of healing that changed everything. I learned how to take care of myself in deep and sustainable ways by using principles of the revolutionary science of Functional Medicine and body-mind wisdom. I learned new, more ennobling and supportive ways of looking at the central stories of my life—stories that I will share with you throughout this book—and my potential for healing. I learned that what I was told was "normal" was wholly unacceptable. I created and adopted a whole new normal, which I am now sharing with you.

MY CALL FOR A NEW PARADIGM OF HEALING

What I've learned through my own healing journey and those of my clients, is that deep, sustainable energy recovery can't be done in the usual, outdated twentieth century way.

We can't do it with conventional medicine—a model of healthcare that's primarily about patching up acute problems.

As a doctor, that was something I didn't come to understand overnight. I heard my clients and their countless stories of disillusionment with the medicine that failed them time and again. Initially I searched for the reasons they and their diseases were special. Why couldn't the great institution of Western medicine help them? But as I listened and learned, I realized the lack of success wasn't about my clients or the uniqueness of their suffering—it was about the medicine they put their faith in.

Conventional medicine is designed quite brilliantly to save lives and address acute symptoms. And make no mistake, for emergency problems, like appendicitis, a heart attack, or broken leg, conventional medicine is the ideal medical model, leading to rapid assessment and essential, often life-saving treatment. But most of our problems aren't emergencies. The conventional acute-care strategy *simply does not work* for most of our health problems and our deeper aspirations for healing.

How Conventional Medicine Can Fall Short:

- by focusing on the quick relief of acute symptoms when most of our problems are chronic, missing the chance to help us on a deeper level to create sustainable, root-cause-level solutions;

- by treating just our symptoms, often with toxic drugs that beget their own problems, leading to unsatisfying results, or worse, greater suffering;

- by offering one-size-fits-all treatment protocols that fail to understand us as unique individuals—and therefore fail *us*;

- by failing to give us the time we need for true understanding, over-simplifying our problems and losing the rich context and complexity of our life stories— leading to incorrect diagnoses and delayed healing;

- by parceling us out on the basis of where we hurt or which organ is in trouble, losing the integration that is the true wisdom of our bodies.

Too often conventional medicine fails to connect with us as human beings or support our innate wisdom about what we each need to heal. By not embracing who we are and our larger stories, this commonplace practice diminishes the possibility for meaningful connection. It's just interaction. Transaction. And usually, dissatisfaction. I found this wholly unsatisfying and unacceptable. It failed me and failed my clients struggling with chronic problems, leaving them without solutions or hope.

Barking Up the Wrong Tree

The prevailing medical model is not an immutable law of nature. It is a *construct of thought*—a belief system, a story—with a set of tools and treatment standards, created by human beings with specific historical and political underpinnings that make it what it is. Its dogma has become entrenched in our culture and accepted as "the truth," and "the way it is," leading to expectations about what the best healthcare is. But it's *a* truth, not *the* truth. It doesn't take the best care of human beings, especially those struggling with persistent fatigue and chronic, complex illness requiring deeper levels of personal agency and wisdom to recover from.

We can do better. To recover our energy and potential, we *must* do better. The real problem with conventional acute-care medicine is not in how it fails us, but with *our expectations* for what it can offer us—we've been barking up the wrong tree! We've got to write a new story of what the best healthcare is, what the best medicine is, and what it takes to live a healing life.

OUR NEW STORY OF HEALING: IT'S IN OUR HANDS

It's clear what we have to do. We've got to call our power back.

To claim our healing, we must embrace the truth that it's within our domain. It's in our hands. Yes, we were *born* to heal. It's our potential. But to activate this potential, we must affirm it. We must claim responsibility for it. We must call our power back from the outside sources we ask to "fix" us. From the "experts" who don't know us as well as we do. Who attempt to define our problems and address our needs with their limited tools and understanding about who we are. We must own the truth that we can change and that we can direct that change to our advantage. We must educate ourselves, learn the skills, find the tools, and create the trusted team of supporters and advisors to guide us as we create our new paradigm of healing.

Yes, you're hearing me right: we must reclaim the idea that we can heal *ourselves*. This is the path I'm asking you to walk with me.

Healing is a Primary Urge of All Nature

We must recall that healing is a primary urge of all nature—all things heal. We see it all around us in landscapes devastated by forest fires, hurricanes, and tornadoes. As annihilation miraculously morphs into new growth and potential. As hopelessness emerges as hope. Inherently a part of the natural world, we have exactly the same potential for rebirth into something we couldn't imagine before. We can passively accept our innate healing trajectory and fall short of our desires and true potential. Or we can *actively* direct this process. We can harness the gifts of nature, of our own biology, to engage and support our healing. But we must claim responsibility for this. We must *own* our healing. We must actively lead the journey of becoming our optimal selves.

So how do we do it? How do we claim this power of ours?

First, We Commit to This Journey

In this book, I'll introduce you to our new roadmap—where you'll see the terrain of your healing life laid out before you. We'll explore the Nine Domains of Healing to see the key elements of energy recovery and healing we'll focus on and direct our actions toward. Each domain is supported by the leading edge science of human potential: epigenetics (how our genetic expression and biology are determined by how we live our lives), neuroplasticity (our brain's enormous potential to change and heal), core systems biology, and body-mind psychology. But before the roadmap, before the bird's eye view of our healing landscape, we've got to open our eyes and commit to this journey.

How?

We show up. We go slow. We pay attention.

Without showing up, going slow, and paying attention, none of our self-care efforts will work. Or if they work, we won't be able to sustain them. They'll get lost in the noise, chaos, and suffering of our lives.

By showing up we may be asked to step out of our comfort zones. Many of us are used to going fast, striving hard, and reaching for the goals out in front of us. What might happen if we show up for *ourselves*? Right here, right now. Will our lives and all the dreams and aspirations we've worked so hard for pass us by?

No. Our lives—our true lives, our healing lives—are right here. In present-moment awareness. Just waiting for us to see—*really* see—and participate. Not fretting about the past or worrying (and planning and striving) about a future that does not yet exist.

Then, through our wide-open eyes, in our present-moment awareness, we clearly see the roadmap and the areas of our lives that most need our attention. We then can call in guidance that makes the most sense to our real lives.

Our New Story of Healing

In this foundational way, we can change our medicine. We can change our lives. We can call our power back by choosing a new story of healing. Our new story of healing includes a roadmap of our choosing that guides our way. Our new story of healing includes tools that fit well in our hands and skills that support our real lives. Our new story of healing is inspired by the authenticity of Life School—our greatest teacher—*ourselves*. Our new story of healing is found by showing up, going slow, and paying attention.

Introductory Exercise to Taste the Path—Practice Being Present

I want you to take a few seconds and pause from reading, just long enough to let go of your thoughts— which by their very nature exist in past or future time—and get into your body, which is inherently linked to the present moment.

Take a deep cleansing belly breath. Breathe into the belly, hold just a second, then let go with an audible sigh. Repeat this several times. With your awareness on your breath, you have entered present time.

Now, let's add a little action. Sit down, and pet and coo over your dog or cat. Smell a rose, slowly inhaling its perfume and let it permeate your whole being. Think of something hilariously funny and let yourself laugh. Lie down on your back (right there on your floor) and let your arms and legs splay out comfortably around you. Feel your whole body against the ground and breathe.

Focus your awareness on your breath and your task. Then come on back.

That was you in present-moment awareness. Not so hard, eh? This is the foundation of all our lessons and practices throughout this book. This is the key to your healing life.

THE PATH—YOUR ROADMAP FOR A HEALING LIFE

This is the journey of our lives, but we do not take it alone. We must engage trusted, valued partners to encourage us, support us, guide us, and give us feedback. And we must come prepared. We urgently need a roadmap for how best to take care of ourselves. We need to see the bird's eye view of the terrain in front of us and choose what we need for ourselves. We need our power back. This is where I can help you.

I am highly trained: I have board certifications in internal medicine and Functional Medicine, and I am a founding diplomate of the pioneering American Board of Holistic Medicine. But my greatest teacher is Life School, what I call the profound lessons of my own experiences as a person, a physician, and a patient, and how I've integrated them with science, cultural wisdom, and experiential knowledge, gleaned from my work with thousands of clients—my true teachers, most of whom discovered their path of healing— over my many years of practicing medicine. From this work, inspired by the innovative science of Functional Medicine, the genius of body-mind wisdom, and my clients' transformational journeys, I've synthesized a roadmap based on our commonalities, which I can't wait to introduce you to.

Our new Nine Domains of Healing roadmap will guide us on a journey that explores our needs and problems as whole people, that offers solutions that go straight to the cause and to the heart of all healing—recovery of our precious energy. You will find our journey is grounded in the fundamental ways we care for ourselves because we know the bones of our healing are in how we call our power back: how we show up, slow down, pay attention, let go, love, balance, sleep, move, eat, think, feel, and live.

We'll take this beautiful journey together. Through me, you are connected to thousands of clients I've worked with and the countless others just like us, ready to step up into the power of their inner wisdom and courage. We'll share and build on our successes. We don't have to reinvent the wheel or make the same mistakes. We know where we're headed: Big Energy. Potential. Wholeness. Healing.

Our new story of healing—our power, our energy, our health—will become the path as well as the prize: the way to our untapped potential.

LAST THOUGHTS—OUR LIVES ARE MIRACLES

Why? Why do we work to heal ourselves?

Because our lives are miracles. Because our true potential, when realized, is a miracle, begets miracles, sees and understands the miracles all around us.

In the end, the greatest miracles are in discovering our true selves, our true potential, and the deep meaning of our lives. Only through deep awareness and recovery of our bodies can these deeper aspects of us be revealed.

I know this all for sure. I see it in all the stories of struggle and transformation that I'm privileged to witness every day in my consultation room. We're all on this hero's journey. We are common people with great, but perhaps untapped courage, strength, and accomplishment. We are not superpeople with superpowers. We are ordinary people deciding to create change in our lives.

It takes great courage to step up to the change that leads to healing. But the heroism and healing seem more commonplace to me now, knowing what I know and have learned from decades of study and experience and knowing how completely accessible deep healing is to even those people who are the most sick and dysfunctional.

It is my hope that this remarkable transformation becomes accessible to everyone, that it becomes more commonplace. That the miraculous becomes commonplace. My hope is that more people will discover the miraculous nature of their lives and how fully accessible it is to each one of us.

This is the ultimate message of this book: that your healing is in your own hands. All you need to recover your energy and vitality is accessible to you, right now. A new roadmap is available to you here, within this book, and healing your body is only the beginning. By nourishing your body and accessing your true power through showing up, going slow, and paying attention, you expand your energy, your strength, and your resilience to live a healing life. And your healing and energy elevates your experience as a human inhabiting a meaningful, purposeful, and extraordinary life.

Your life is a miracle.

Chapter One

FIRST, CLAIM YOUR HEALING

Healing is ours. Our birthright. The primary urge of all nature. But we must claim it as our own. No one else can do this for us. Our healing, our wholeness, our potential rests squarely in our own hands.

This is power. This is our power. This is the promise of our amazing humanness.

It all begins with a simple decision. A "yes," softly spoken, perhaps tentatively at first, that precedes the next "yes," and the next. Or bellowed out from the gut, ready to release suffering, ripe for this journey of self-discovery and healing.

But each decision, however soft or booming, is singularly powerful. Each one a beginning. Each one staking its claim. Each one tenacious and alive with intention.

Let us share this common bond of truth seeking and thirst for claiming what is ours—our story, our power—by walking this path together.

We know where we're headed: Energy. Potential. Wholeness. Healing.

START HERE—TELL YOUR STORY

The first act of reclaiming our power is telling our story of becoming well. We say it, imagine it, and thereby breathe life into it. That's how we can begin to reclaim the power we may have given away to the experts who we believe know more than we do. The power we may have subdued through our resistance to change, our fear of failure, or our beliefs of unworthiness and not having time. The power we may have lost sight of, buried in our fatigue, our overwhelm, or our suffering. The power that is still there, ripe for the taking.

So, let's start with your story of becoming well. *Your* story. Because this is *your* life, *your* journey, *your* potential. Only you can tell this story. Only you can name your hopes, desires, and goals—your destination. This is where your hero's journey (yes, you are a hero!) to Big Energy recovery and healing begins.

Tell Your Story of Becoming Well

Even if you feel totally tanked, hopeless, disbelieving, lost, or pessimistic about your future, you can still tell your story. Let's take this first crucial step together.

Write your new life story. Your healing story. Your story of becoming well. This will just be your first draft. But it's the all-important beginning where you stake your claim to a better future. Where you say *yes* to this journey. Where you begin to build the mind pathways of hope that support and nourish you.

First, Breathe

Breathe deeply in and out and let it all go. Let your breath guide you into your body. Soften your judgments. Soften your disbelief. Come along on this journey with us. Just breathe.

Declare Your "Yes"

Say yes.

Yes to healing. Yes to a better future. Yes to opening the door to possibilities—even if just a crack.

Say yes in any way you feel inspired. A single word. Yes. Or long flowing sentences. Yes, yes, yes!

List Your Goals and Desires

Find a blank piece of paper or use the margins of this book. Don't worry, this is not a quiz. This is for you—no one else will see this unless you choose to share. Write down your goals and desires. Forget the complete sentences, punctuation, and flowing prose. Ditch the perfectionism and just write.

What do you, in your deepest heart of hearts, want to achieve? What are your goals for healing? This journey must be about *you*. It doesn't matter what anyone else would have you do or aspire to. This is *your* life story. Claim it now. (Hint: it is not necessary to diagnose yourself or know anything at all about *what* needs to be healed. This is simply you stating what you want to achieve: To have more energy? To reach your potential? To feel like yourself again? To be able to compete in your first ironman? To be able to work again or go back to school? See what I'm asking you to do?)

Now, Imagine You've Achieved Those Goals

What does your healing life look like? Can you see or feel differences in your world? What do you feel like in your body, mind, and spirit? What are you doing? What do you look like? Who else is there with you at your side? What's possible? Now that you've imagined successfully achieving these first goals, are there more that come to mind? Perhaps goals you never dreamed were possible?

Congratulations! You've just called your power back. You may not feel it yet. You may detect just a trickle of hope. You may sense a bit of strength rise up from your gut. This is only the beginning.

Once upon a time there was a hero/heroine named [insert your name here], and they began a wondrous journey . . .

OUR BEAUTIFUL ENERGY ROADMAP—THE NINE DOMAINS OF HEALING

You've called your power back by envisioning your destination. Now what do you need?

Well, on any worthwhile journey it helps to have a mentor (me!), tools (we've got lots of tools to explore and put to use throughout this book), fellow travelers (we're all here with you!), and a roadmap with suggestions for directions that we choose based on where we are and where we want to be. A nuanced roadmap that knows the best path isn't always a straight line from point A to point B. Our paths through the terrain of our healing will be different. For each of us, our paths may loop back, revisiting areas we've already been, or exploring side paths of interest.

Throughout this book, that roadmap will be the Nine Domains of Healing. These nine domains are the keys to reclaiming your power. Each domain explores, teaches, and guides you through a different foundational aspect of the healing life. They merge the great traditions of human science—state of the art physiology, Functional Medicine systems biology, body-mind psychology, and integrative spirituality—with wisdom from Life School: healing insights that cross cultures and contain the knowledge and observations from my consultation room, acquired from nearly thirty years of working with people just like you.

Each of the Nine Domains of Healing reminds us of our deep potential for growth and healing in every aspect of our lives through the core science of epigenetics and neuroplasticity.[1] Each domain invites you to call your power back to an essential aspect of yourself, to create your healing life.

---

[1] Epigenetics and neuroplasticity are well proven scientific concepts that make clear our potential for profound change and healing through every aspect of how we live our lives. Excellent resources for further reading: Norman Doidge, MD. *The Brain That Changes Itself.* 2007; and Kenneth R. Pelletier. *Change Your Genes, Change Your Life: Creating Optimal Health with the New Science of Epigenetics.* 2018.

The Nine Domains of Healing

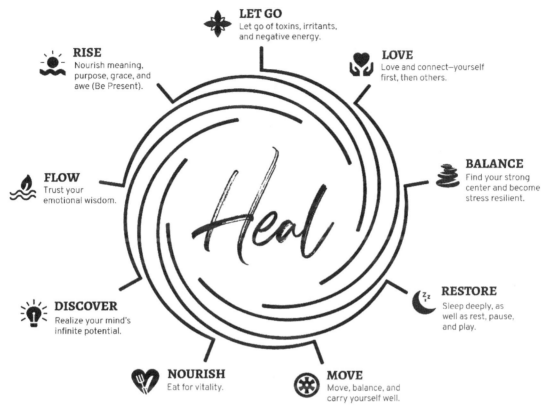

LET GO
Let go of toxins, irritants, and negative energy.

RISE
Nourish meaning, purpose, grace, and awe (Be Present).

LOVE
Love and connect—yourself first, then others.

FLOW
Trust your emotional wisdom.

BALANCE
Find your strong center and become stress resilient.

DISCOVER
Realize your mind's infinite potential.

RESTORE
Sleep deeply, as well as rest, pause, and play.

NOURISH
Eat for vitality.

MOVE
Move, balance, and carry yourself well.

© 2018 Karyn Shanks MD

As you can see, the Nine Domains of Healing roadmap is multi-layered, with one domain flowing into the next, all integrated as one whole—just as *we* are.

This is the healing roadmap that respects us as the people who we are. Multifaceted. Complex. Not needing to be "fixed," but empowered. Not being told what to do or where we "need" to go but shown the lay of the land so we can choose for ourselves—with perhaps messy and stressful lives, but lives that are also beautiful, heroic, and uniquely ours.

This Nine Domains of Healing roadmap supports our innate strength and wisdom, however unrealized it may be in our fatigue or suffering. It will serve as our guide, and source of encouragement and inspiration. It will be in our hands to help us as we take this intuitive journey of our lives, explore our problems and struggles, and find the resources we need.

Yes, this beautiful energy roadmap, the Nine Domains of Healing, will accompany us all the way on this big journey of ours to creating a healing life. Allow me to introduce you to each domain.

LET GO

To Create Space for Healing, Let Go of Toxins, Irritants, and Negative Energy

As we let go, clear out, and slow down we create space for healing and energy recovery to occur, knowing we can't bring in the new until the old is reckoned with. Letting go—of the toxins and irritants that make us sick; the habits that don't nourish us; the incessant distractions that consume our precious time, attention, and energy; the negative energy of people and old stories that hold us back— brings in new life, new hope, new potential. It literally frees up energy and space for healing to occur.

LOVE

Love and Connect (Yourself First, Then Others)

With our newly created space, we let the love in—the love that is our destination, our purpose, and our path. We thrive when love flows into our lives. But though love is all around us, accessible to us all, we can lose our connection to it. In our fatigue and suffering we can forget our worthiness for love. In the domain of *LOVE* we explore the necessity of loving ourselves first, then extending our hearts out to others, creating the circle of love that is the strength of our humanity and the source of our healing.

BALANCE

Find Your Strong Center and Become Stress Resilient

Having created space and welcomed love, we now can find, nurture, and fortify our center. Our center is *us*—our wise inner self, our strength, and, like a compass rose, our internal place of balance. From this core of our being we take on the challenges, struggles, joys, and the daily chores.

In the domain of *BALANCE*, we explore how to create a strong center to support our dynamic vitality. We'll learn to bolster the biological energy that sustains our center—the stress response (the physiology of energy and the power of our core) and the brain-thyroid-adrenal-mitochondrial (BTAM) energy operating system. We'll learn to savor how it fuels us in the face of all that life brings us.

RESTORE

Sleep Deeply, as well as Pause, Rest, and Play

As we embrace the challenges of our lives and create our strong center, we must also rest. Sleep is powerful medicine and a magical, mysterious time that allows us to power down, repair, replenish, and renew, providing the deepest restoration of energy and wellbeing available to us. We'll learn how sleep is the boss—it can't be hacked, passed over, substituted for, or shorted without devastating consequences. We'll explore the ways that deep restorative sleep, as well as pause, rest, and play, are available to us all.

MOVE

Move, Balance, and Carry Yourself Well

We were born to move—to survive, to seek, to play, and to love. Established by our ancestors long ago, there is an exquisite genetic relationship between movement and our biology, our biology and function, our function and wellbeing. This central biology was calibrated to operate optimally at our ancestors' level of activity—on the move constantly to meet their subsistence needs. But our immediate survival no longer depends on such a hard working life. Many of us hardly move at all.

We need our bodies strong, stable, nimble, and ready to engage. And we must be *in* our bodies. For this we must learn to show up for them, unraveling old entrenched habits and creating new ones through how we move, balance, and carry ourselves well.

NOURISH

Eat for Vitality

You knew we'd get to this, didn't you? Yes, we literally *are* what we eat. The molecules we eat become *us*, for better or worse. Our food turns on and off our genes to make us who we are—to fuel our energy and support all function. Or, put the brakes on our healing. We get to choose at this powerful control point of our biology.

Food is a foundational, nonnegotiable part of the journey to our energy recovery and healing. We will share powerful stories of healing through food, and suggest a compelling, science-based, and thoroughly street-tested roadmap for your own nutritional healing.

DISCOVER

Realize Your Mind's Infinite Potential (Claim Your True Life Stories)

Our minds are our greatest tools and advisors but understanding them is never simple. Our brains were designed to keep us alive by telling stories. Our stories have great power—they can strengthen us, or they can stop us soundly in our tracks. We must honor the stories of our lives and how they may have served us at one time and helped us survive. But it's time to scrutinize our stories for their value and truth as we step into our power and potential. We must release the toxic stories that hold us back.

We'll explore the science of neural networks and neuroplasticity—the biology of stories—and the promise of our brains to change to create new, intentional, powerful healing stories.

FLOW

Trust Your Emotional Wisdom (Find Your Truth)

Here we explore the wisdom of our deepest, wisest selves—our emotional genius. We learn to honor our emotions, feelings, and sensations of our bodies as pure unadulterated feedback about the truth of us—who we are, what's going on in our environments, the people around us, and the conditions of our lives. Taught by our culture to cut ourselves off from our emotions in favor of our more rational minds (and stories), we may be entering unfamiliar and uncomfortable territory. Yes, we'll squirm, but we must step into our fear to claim the raw truth of our emotional wisdom.

RISE

Nourish Meaning, Purpose, Grace, and Awe (Be Present)

Finally, we rise. We rise in small ways—with each intention, each decision, each step, each small victory, each celebration of ourselves and our commitment to our healing life. And we rise big as our self-care opens space, fuels energy, and nudges (or catapults) us into our potential. Because our energy, clarity, and practiced intention to ourselves, our bodies, this moment, and the beauty of the world all around us anchors us in present time. This presence is our ultimate healing, and it reveals the path as well as the prize—the meaning, purpose, grace, and awe of our entire lives.

HOW TO PACK FOR YOUR HEALING JOURNEY

You've called your power back and envisioned your destination. You see the terrain—and the many possibilities for the way there. You have the roadmap in your hands that will accompany you and support you in your travels. You feel the anticipation for the journey. You're scared, but you've made the commitment—you've said *yes*.

This healing that you've asked for is a journey. And like all journeys, you must come prepared. Just as you'd need to pack your toothbrush for a trip, healing requires that you pack and know where to find the parts of yourself that are essential to this journey.

And you've got to travel light. You must also know what to leave behind—those things that weigh you down, distract you, and get in the way of your progress.

First, Hope

We're wired to know that tomorrow will be a better day than today. We *know* this. Hope is that opening in our thinking that something better is possible—that *healing* is possible. We may not see the healing or know what it is, but we believe in the possibilities.

Harness the Extraordinary Power of Practice

The story of your healing is what you *do*.

In other words, we must *live* this journey. Healing, wholeness, energy recovery, potential—all that we aspire to—are in what we practice every day. Not what we plan, think about, or ponder. They're what we live. Right now.

Let Go of the Need to Be *All Ready*

When are we ever ready—*really* ready—for jumping over the precipice of big change into the abyss of the unknown? Isn't that just what it feels like? Even the new food plan, gym, or yoga class feels scary. That very first walking across the threshold into our new lives—into change—is so hard!

In spite of not feeling ready, we all have the capacity to be brave, to be optimistic, to have hope, and to commit. We can all do these hard things even when we're scared and uncertain about the outcome.

Let Go of the Need to Be Perfect

We must not allow our drive for unattainable perfection sabotage our efforts to heal. The path to perfection always leads to failure and disappointment. Perfection is the impossible urge to control all possible variables of our lives—to avoid mistakes and failures. We must cherish the adventure of our journey, mistakes and failures and all, and trust that all outcomes born from our best efforts always guide us in the direction that is right for *us*.

Let Go of the Need to Know What Happens Next

Uncertainty makes us squirm, doesn't it? But the unexpected is the only certainty in this life. Imagine the smashing, exhilarating things that happen to us that we'd miss if we didn't take risks. We must be brave and embrace the responsibility of making choices and taking action—they all involve risk. Uncertainty will inevitably lead us to roadblocks and setbacks, but also to the many joys of the evolution of our healing and spectacular life.

Let Go of the Need for Permission

To embark on steps to heal, the mature mind only needs permission from itself, not from the "experts," loved ones, or members of the tribe. We must reclaim this personal power for ourselves and let go of the judgment and shame that get in our way—to imagine, to hear our inner guidance, to decide, and to take decisive action. Because we say so.

Let Go of the Need to Have It Easy

You didn't really think it would be easy, did you? It's true, we get to glide sometimes, but that's our reward for hard work. While we must learn the art of pause, rest, and play, we must also embrace how a life worth living is a call to challenge. And, as we'll learn, challenge creates our strength. But what's harder? A bit of practice each day as we take one step at a time, one moment at a time, to claim our power and healing? Or displacing our energy into resisting our call and fearful imaginings about what our challenges ask of us, and going nowhere?

Let Go of the Fear of Deprivation

Yes, we've all experienced loss and deprivation associated with changes we've invited into our lives. We grieve the loss of our very worst habits—the comfort, the solace, the rewards. And we feel the agony of our cravings, longings, and unfulfilled desires. But deprivation is a short-term discomfort for long-term gains that we can manage. We'll explore tools to help us with this.

Let Go of the Need for One-Size-Fits-All Solutions to Our Problems

We're not all the same. Life is not that simple. We'll no longer accept being inconveniences to those who try to stick us in their box, use their one-size-fits-all protocols to "fix" us, and prescribe treatments that don't fit us—and don't work! On this journey we'll explore *your* unique story and *your* unique needs to achieve sustainable solutions to *your* unique problems. Yes, this journey is a celebration of *you*!

FINALLY, HEALING IS NOT ALWAYS CURING

Healing is our innate trajectory. The primary impulse of all living things is to heal. Look at the natural world. Earth destroyed by fire or volcanic flow will soon sprout new trees and flowers. The waters flow again, and the animals return. A new landscape takes the place of what once looked like total devastation. And it never looks like what we'd expect—what we fear we'll have to settle for. The scars are still there—the deep crags and crevices, the upended rocks, the deep valleys. But look at how our perceptions change, as time heals, as the remarkable beauty of healing takes hold. The earth's potential for rebirth is not only unpredictable, but also miraculous, jaw dropping, awe-inspiring. Nature does not settle for cures.

We're just the same. We may look for cures. But what we get instead, when we actively pursue our healing, when we work the Nine Domains of Healing roadmap, is something far greater. We may not be cured—we may have scars, disabilities, and vulnerabilities that will need our lifelong attention—but we get our own true, perhaps unpredictable, jaw dropping, and awe-inspiring potential. Consider the phenomenal life of Stephen

Hawking—never cured of his disease, confined to a wheelchair and unable to speak, but nonetheless lived a brilliant healing life and soared into the stratosphere!

Curing is a story that assumes a particular outcome about not being sick, no longer having that "disease," or no longer suffering. But healing is much bigger than that. Curing is inherently limited in its scope. Healing opens us to the possibilities that may be beyond our wildest dreams. If we release the story of curing, while lovingly, reverently caring for ourselves, where does that land us? Healing. Wholeness. Potential.

LAST THOUGHTS: WELCOME TO MY TRAVEL COMPANIONS

I am so grateful you are here with me. That we get to take this remarkable journey together. And that you've shown up for yourself in this beautiful and powerful way. Your energy and vitality are necessary for you to live and express the potential that is within you. And beyond yourself, *the world needs your potential*. Whoever you are, whatever your strengths, whatever your ambitions—however grand, simple, or commonplace—the world needs the very best of you now.

Your healing journey is vital.

And it is within your reach. Right here. Right now. With us.

Chapter Two

LET GO

To Create Space for Healing,
Let Go of Toxins, Irritants, and Negative Energy

The journey is long. The journey is arduous. The journey is for our lives.

And yet, wait . . . what's that? Ah, yes . . . we can lay down our vigilance and worry. For the primary urge of all nature is to heal—it's the wisdom of our own tired and imperfect bodies.

Healing is us. It's in us, not needing our permission. We need only breathe, and trust, and listen as our bodies whisper (or scream) their requests.

And when we're still, and present—believing in the miracle within us—we create space. Space for healing. Space for evolution. Space for the energy we seek.

MANDY'S GENIUS

My client Mandy floored me with her insights about what she needed to heal in a deep and sustainable way. Her simple genius helped me clarify the necessary starting point for all our healing: Let Go.

When Mandy came to see me for the first time just over a year ago, she was a mess. She'd been suffering from deep fatigue, muscle and joint aches, brain fog, high anxiety, persistent diarrhea, abdominal pain, and facial nerve pain. Her symptoms had started the previous year, shortly after cleaning up the black mold discovered in the basement of her house. She remediated the moldy materials herself, deconstructing contaminated walls and floors, and overseeing the placement of new materials.

Extensive evaluation of her lifelong health history and review of her current problems and lab work revealed that she was sick from an overwhelming load of toxicity—but not just from mold. She was highly stressed, anxious, slept poorly, and made little time to tend to her own needs. She was sick from toxins within the mold as well as toxins from her internal environment: increased intestinal permeability, food sensitivities, imbalanced gut flora, and deficiencies of key nutrients needed to clear toxins from her body.

She enthusiastically embarked on a comprehensive treatment plan that included a strict anti-inflammatory-intensive nutrition food plan[2], supplementation of essential nutrients, probiotics and digestive enzymes, a strict sleep hygiene program, and moderate exercise. She was able to dive in full on because, as a schoolteacher, she had the summer off to focus extra time on herself, and she was anxious to feel better.

She flourished. By the time I saw her back in the office six weeks later, all of her symptoms were gone except for the facial nerve pain. Mandy was energetic, vibrant, and full of life.

But then school started back up in the fall, and the stresses and time constraints that come with being a very busy kindergarten teacher and mom challenged her. She started eating comfort foods—sugar, gluten, and dairy (her worst offenders as inflammation triggers)—which were all too easily accessible in the teachers' lounge. She found herself going to bed later and later. She could not sustain her exercise regimen, and she began spending increasing amounts of time on social media after work—an easy way to relax and decompress after a busy, stressful day, but hard to put down.

All her symptoms returned. They weren't as severe as they had been, since she kept up with much of her earlier regimen, but she was disappointed to lose the vibrancy she had enjoyed for several months. Of course, she wondered what *she* had done wrong.

---

[2] *Gut-Immune Restoration Intensive Nutrition (GRIN)* food plan, discussed in chapter seven: NOURISH.

In our most recent meeting, she came in with a list. She had thought it through very carefully. She wanted to feel well again and was very clear about what aspects of self-care would get her there. There was no doubt what had led to her complete recovery before. Her challenge now was to sustain her healing in the face of the school year stresses. Because she had paid attention, she learned from her "failure." She had to create the space, time, and practice for her healing.

She handed me her list of three things:

1. **Get more sleep to open up space for restoration and repair.** She planned to start with fifteen extra minutes per night and work up gradually to an extra hour, then to an hour and a half each night.

2. **Stop time wasting to open up space for other self-care tasks.** She put strict limits on the time spent on social media, which had become a huge time suck. A little bit is good—engagement with friends, enjoyment of articles and funny stories. But too much left no time for the self-care she needed.

3. **Begin a meditation practice to open space in her mind, relax, and relieve anxiety.** She had begun using a meditation app we'd discussed at an earlier visit, setting it for just fifteen minutes each morning and meditating before doing anything else. She was already feeling the expansion it was creating, leading to reduced stress and anxiety, and helping her feel a more positive and hopeful outlook as she started each day.

This woman nailed it! She intuitively recognized the need to create space in her life for healing to take place in a sustainable way by letting go of the things that held her back. Using her own insights into the demands of her body, in her very own words, she beautifully articulated her hierarchy of needs.

And that is the whole point of this chapter—this crucial first domain of healing: *we must let go*. We must let go of the toxicity, irritants, and negative energy to make room for the healing—to make room for the resources, time, and energy for the active self-care we need.

WE ALL KNOW WHAT TOXICITY IS

Everyone knows what toxicity feels like. It's the sickening headache that comes on when we've gotten stuck behind an old beater on the highway, belching smoke into our path. It's the awful feeling of being in the same room with someone who is needy, manipulative, and resentful who slowly sucks the life from us before we realize what's happening. It's being overwhelmed by too much clutter, distraction, time pressure, or excessive engagement with negative news and social media. It's too much sugar, too much alcohol, or not enough sleep. It saps our strength, our energy, our vigor, and our time. We're depleted. Unwell. Not ourselves. Toxic!

In this chapter we'll create space for healing by letting go of the common obstacles that hold us back: the toxins, irritants, negative energy, distractions, and time wasters that put the brakes on our healing life. For some of you, letting go is all you'll need to unlock a wellspring of energy and potential. Letting go brings in new life, new hope, new possibilities. It literally frees up energy for healing to occur.

Letting go is also realizing you don't have to do this alone. The space you create invites wisdom into your life, opening room for it to live, breathe, and become your tangible reality. Wisdom from your inner self and from sources bigger than you, whatever you conceive them to be—nature, God, the universe—all help you flourish when you give them room to join you.

Letting go is trusting that healing is a primary urge of all nature. All things heal. This healing can be passively observed with diminished effect or actively directed for life-changing impact. To unleash that healing and receive the immense gifts of nature to engage and support your healing, you must first create space.

RECOGNIZING LIFE TOXICITY

Letting go is the easiest, most accessible, and liberating part of our healing journey. The first step is learning to recognize the life toxins that hurt us—then let them go. And when necessary, we won't just let go, we'll eject them fiercely from our lives! While this is not necessarily hard work, some of these life toxins are covert. So we have to show up, go slow, and pay attention to detect them and really see how they operate in our lives. You're probably thinking right now about some of the toxic and negative things holding you back. Resolve to send them packing!

Toxic Stories about Our Healing

I can't . . .
I don't have time . . .
Who am I to . . . ?

These three stories—these few brief words used as preambles to your self-assessment—are toxic. They're excuses. They slam the brakes on healing every single time.

You fill in the blanks. Whatever you put there is a story. These are your personal narratives about what's holding you back. They may be *your* truth—*a* truth—but not *the* truth.

To create space for healing, these stories must go.

I can—I am—I'll show you.
I make time—I clear out clutter and distraction and reveal the abundance of time I have.
I am worthy.

In chapter eight, we'll explore these potentially crushing stories and how to change them in great depth. But now, right now, change a few simple words as you re-read these lines. Whether you believe them or not, change them. They will grow.

Guilt, Shame, and Judgment

Among the most powerful, emotional, and destructive stories we can tell ourselves are those involving guilt, shame, and judgment. Know right now in your core—no matter what you've been told, what you believe, or how you feel—guilt, shame, and judgment have no place in healing and a healthy life. And yet here they are, perched on our shoulders. Blaming us for the predicament we're in, for how we've failed, how we're not enough, how we can't keep up, how we're not tough enough, how we've succumbed to the need to focus on ourselves when so many others need our time and attention. If only we could do it "right," or do it like everyone else does. Or if we were just rich enough, lucky enough, smart enough, or could find just the right pill or treatment we could heal ourselves. Sound familiar?

Guilt, shame, and judgment are as toxic as any cesspool of chemicals. They can even be worse, because they are insidious stories that we often don't see until they stop us in our tracks, cloud our awareness and wisdom and weaken us in the face of the important work we have ahead of us.

The antidotes for these toxic feelings are self-love and compassion. They energize our work to let go of what harms us. They lay bare the falsehood of the guilt, shame, and judgment we inflict on ourselves for not living the "ideal" life, for clinging to old ways and habits we know are not good for us, or for trying to change and failing. Acts of self-love and compassion supercharge our intentions and energize our actions as we move into a new and better future. They let in the wisdom and guidance we need to navigate our new healing path.

But even armed with self-love and compassion, our task to dismantle guilt, shame, and judgment is not easy. They are long used, well-worn emotions with disempowering stories to explain them. They become default pathways for our minds to understand our experiences. They pop up and smack us between the eyes before we even realize they're there. Many of us don't see guilt, shame, and judgment for what they are—we accept their false truths and marinate in the lies they tell us about ourselves. Nothing shuts us down and gets us stuck so completely.

So we need to take action. Realize that self-love and compassion are active, not passive. They are not what we *feel*, but what we *do*. In fact, at the start, we don't have to feel them at all. We may not be able to. Feeling self-love and compassion may be too hard right now. That's okay. *Feeling love is not necessary to begin the practice.* But beginning the practice opens the room for it to grow and the feelings to come.

So, begin here: look honestly and see how you judge yourself for your own suffering. How you carry the guilt and shame of it. And consider a better way, by becoming the compassionate witness—the champion—of yourself.

Why Do We Blame Ourselves for Being Sick?

It seems counterintuitive. People don't consciously *choose* to become sick, depleted, or to suffer. But still, we blame ourselves for our own suffering. I hear these stories every day from my clients: The hopelessness and sense of personal failure after years of chronic pain and fatigue and not finding the answers. The self-reproach for failing yet another food plan. The guilt and shame for asking for help. The total self-neglect in favor of the needs of everyone else.

We've been misled by the belief that self-care is selfish. Much to the contrary, failure to care for ourselves leads us to depletion and remaining stuck in illness. But because we've been taught to be stoic, we don't ask for help, instead silently "soldiering on" in spite of our suffering.

Many of us have been told by our doctors, the "experts," that there is "nothing wrong." Our suffering and fatigue persist, making it hard to remain hopeful and positive about what we can do to create a better future for ourselves. Through it all, we struggle with our worth: who are we to expect healing or ask for help from others? Further, we're scared about the uncertainty of the change required to move us out of illness. What effort will be required of us? What will it cost us? Where will the change we ask for lead us?

How to Become the Compassionate Witness to Neutralize the Toxicity of Guilt, Shame, and Judgment

Suffering is not a character flaw. To heal, we must let go of the blame and judgment and consider another story. A truer story. A heroic one. Your story. We'll rewrite the old story and create a more compassionate one together.

To begin the healing process wherever you are on your journey (in the depths of illness, exhausted, suffering, or just tweaking and optimizing your health), you must be the witness to yourself. Instead of telling your story with all the judgments inside your own brain, pretend that you are a caring outsider and tell your story as it is right now, without judgment, just love.

Suspend all blame. Become the compassionate witness. Bless yourself (I don't mean this in a religious way, but simply as an expression of love and acceptance for how things are right in this moment). Bless your body, just as it is. Bless your difficult emotions, which bring you wisdom about what needs to change. Bless your struggles, which will bear such delicious fruit. Bless the future and potential you perhaps can't see at this moment.

I want you to have compassion for yourself even in your pain, your suffering, your overwhelm, your energy wipeout. Even in your tired and depleted state, you are a unique and very special soul, totally worthy of love, compassion, and understanding, both from yourself and from others. Sophisticated as we can be with our understanding of the biochemistry, structure, and function of healing—with all our brilliant books, plans, strategies, and solutions—none of them mean a thing without compassion and love for ourselves.

The smallest shifts in our thinking and behavior can lead to deep and lasting change within our minds. Neuroscience shows us that all thought and action leads to anatomical and functional changes within our brains—nothing is ever hardwired in. Positive thoughts and actions lead to positive changes that are real, that grow, that transform what can happen in our lives.[3] We can absolutely, profoundly heal with the smallest acts of compassion and self-love.

Exercise: Self-Love and Compassion Can Be in the Small Things We Do

Let's take a quick break to practice being the compassionate witness to ourselves. While it may sound impossible to you right now, it's really quite simple—follow along with us.

------

[3] We'll dive deeper into a discussion about neural networks and the promise of neuroplasticity in chapter eight: DISCOVER.

Imagine yourself totally tanked. Energy gone. Motivation lost. Creative energy squashed. In bed and unable to move. Just be there. Have compassion for yourself as someone who in this moment is not capable of much of anything. See if you can let go of all self-judgment. Just for this moment, see yourself with love, just as you would a small child or an animal needing you to support and not judge them.

There. This infinitesimally small act of kindness to yourself when at your lowest point is the practice of love. It's seeing yourself, and your condition, as you are, through the lens of compassion and kindness, without the negative and self-condemning stories that often accompany feeling depleted and out of gas. This small shift, practiced every day, will create a neural network—a story—that unlocks your potential for healing. That's all it takes.

The Negative Energy of Toxic People

"We have not come into this exquisite world to hold ourselves hostage from love.

Run, my dear, from anything that may not strengthen your precious budding wings,

Run like hell, my dear, from anyone likely to put a sharp knife into the sacred, tender vision of your beautiful heart."

—Hafiz (*Sufi poet, 1310-1390*)

When in the company of people who don't love, honor, and support us, we suffer. When we surround ourselves with people who bring us down—who whine and complain, who need and take but don't give back, who manipulate and criticize, or who are "nice" but don't tell us the truth—we're in trouble. These people and their negative energy suck our souls.

To heal, we must protect ourselves from the toxicity and negative energy of the people in our lives. They can exhaust, deplete, and harm us every bit as much—if not more—as toxic chemicals and bad food. They're poison.

Learning who these people are is not an advanced skill. Even young children innately know the people they're safe with, want to hang out with, or whom they need to get away from. They know how to say "no." And so do we. But, as adults, we've become more practiced at being "nice," neglecting our inner guidance in favor of getting along, or being the "good" daughter, sister, friend, or coworker. But nice isn't truth. Nice may kill you.

When you are confronted with toxic people in your life, I'm here to tell you, like the words of Hafiz, to run like hell. You deserve the love and support of every single person you choose to have in your inner circle. The rest must go. Be careful and savvy about your friends. You know who the good ones are. They're the ones who celebrate you. They're never discouraging or underhanded.

This is hard stuff. It's hard to let go of the toxic people in our lives who we've belonged to for so long. It's hard to set boundaries and not know what the outcome will be. Will we lose them altogether? Will we belong to no one?

By definition, creating personal protective boundaries separates us from others. That can't help but set off alarm signals within our brains, which are wired to protect our social connectedness. We have to accept that as something that isn't bad. To set boundaries we must be willing to stand strong and understand that we are opening space for greater belonging. Opening space for us to be our true selves. Opening space to hear the small quiet voice of truth within. Opening space for others like us to find us and come into our lives.

This ability to stand strong as our authentic selves and protect ourselves from toxic relationships leads to what author Brené Brown calls "true belonging" in her book, *Braving the Wilderness: The Quest for True Belonging and the Courage to Stand Alone*. True belonging is the strength and authenticity we carry inside us. By rising up to this and eliminating the toxic people in our lives, we create space for our true selves and people who are more like us. In this place, as Brown describes, "we belong everywhere and nowhere."

Our strength is in belonging to ourselves first. In this we create space for love.

Distraction

Distraction—so ubiquitous, so available, so enticing—sucks the life out of us.

Here's the deal. Our brains were not designed to multitask with any competence or efficiency, despite common belief to the contrary. Study after study has shown that we do our best when we focus on doing just one thing at a time. As we divide our attention between multiple tasks, our efficiency and accuracy fall off precipitously no matter how seemingly simple the tasks are. The result? Our performance becomes inferior to what we're capable of. Our stress increases. Distractions that persist lead to an internal state of alarm. So we end up stressed, overwhelmed, and less competent.

And it gets worse! In addition to leaving us stressed, these distractions *sap our time*, which makes us feel like there aren't enough hours in the day. That leaves us with no time to heal. No time to do the things that would really nourish us.

Giving ourselves permission to focus on just one thing at a time makes us smarter and better, while allowing us to slow down, relax, and claim the time we need to live our healing lives.

Technological Distraction

I love technology. I mean, what did we do without Google and Amazon? Or cell phones and texting? Or laptops and clouds and wireless networks? These are all incredible conveniences. And isn't social media a great way to stay connected and share information? If only we didn't have so much trouble turning it off. We all know the temptation to check those notifications on our mobile devices, keeping our finger on the pulse of what's happened now and who's entering the conversation.

There's no question technology has made our lives more convenient in huge ways. When I was in medical school, before the age of the internet, I had to go to the library every time I wanted to research a single question. I searched the card catalogue, pulled volumes of journals from the shelves, and painstakingly read through them. Now I pull up an electronic PubMed search in seconds. Mind blowing!

It's great when we use all these things to our advantage. But it's easy to get lulled into the sense that we can get more done *all at once*. Truth is: we can't. If you think you can, chances are you're not performing your tasks all that well.

We easily overconsume technology, making ourselves less focused on one thing, overly stimulated, overtired, and distracted. While we think we're more connected, we actually become disconnected from what we care about—people, experiences, and the moment right here in front of us. And we're more stressed-out than ever.

Case in point: cell phone use while driving, an intersection of our nation's favorite pastimes. The scientific literature on cell phone use while driving is clear and alarming: our driving performance while talking on the phone—*handheld as well as hands-free*—is on par with driving drunk. An elegant study by Strayer and colleagues at the University of Utah compared distracted drivers using their phones to intoxicated drivers. When both driving conditions and time spent driving were controlled, the distracted drivers' (using both handheld and hands-free devices) impairments were as profound as those associated with driving drunk.[4] It is currently estimated that at least half of all car accidents are related to cell phone use. Most everyone ignores the warnings not to use cell phones while driving, even people I consider to be smart. They don't believe the data or don't want to know—knowing would mean giving up this addiction.

Driving is a complex, dynamic task. In many respects driving already is multitasking, making it a unique challenge. How many of us have had the experience of not remembering our drive for many miles when we have been deep in thought or engrossed in conversation? How many near misses have we experienced when our attention was diverted for just a second? Now, throw talking on the phone into the mix. Our brains prioritize the phone conversation over attention to our environment. The result? Our responses are delayed, we are less alert, and much more apt to make mistakes or act to avoid the mistakes of other drivers. Whether you want to believe this or not, it is irrefutably true.

Bottom line? When you drive, just drive. When you connect with others, just connect. Claim responsibility for the stress you create in yourself as well as others. Be present. Release stress. Create time.

---

[4] DL Strayer, et al. *A Comparison of the Cell Phone Driver and the Drunk Driver. Human Factors.* 2006 Summer; 48(2): 381-91.

Negative Information—Distraction from What's Good

This really is a very good world, a beautiful world, a magical and enchanting world in so many ways. If I let myself, I get to experience one magnificent part of it after another—from the warm comfy bed I wake up in every morning, to the birds and trees outside my meditation window, to the amazing heroic people I meet throughout my day. Your life is filled with these miracles too.

But it's easy to miss and forget all this when we marinate ourselves in the barrage of negative information so well concentrated for us by the media. As we'll discuss in more detail in chapter eight, the human brain gloms onto fear and darkness as a survival mechanism. The news outlets, wanting to sell news, know this. All good intentions aside, we ultimately receive the very worst and cataclysmic of what makes up our world, making it easy to forget that it's actually quite wonderful out there. Yes, there's bad stuff too—pain, sickness, and injustice that we need to be aware of. We can't stay completely insulated and maintain our humanity. But too much distraction by negative information is toxic, stressful, and depletes us.

The best way to manage this barrage of negative information is to place limits on your exposure to it.

How to Reduce the Toxicity of Negative Information

- Avoid starting your day with news or negative information. Our psyches are more permeable and less defensible to the onslaught of negativity first thing in the day.

- Place limits on overall daily exposure to news—Isn't once a day enough?

- Take news fasts. Go for periods of time—a week, two weeks—without any news exposure at all.

- Turn off all news notifications on your phone.

- Take care to receive your news from fair, balanced, and legitimate sources to avoid dishonesty and toxicity. Everyone knows which news outlets serve up news that isn't real—they're fear, hate, and lie mongers who create poison, not news.

- Make sure to balance every moment you spend consuming news with consideration of what you appreciate in this world and in your life. Your neural networks of gratitude need stoking too.

Clutter—Environmental Distraction

Clutter in our personal environments commands our senses—we can't help but see it, possibly trip over it, and not find what we're looking for. It's a lot like multitasking. Our sensory perception of those piles of stuff and dirt and mess needs space and processing within our brains. We feel this as distraction, low energy, inability to focus and concentrate, procrastination, inefficiency, a sense of internal chaos. Who hasn't felt the cleansing, freeing feeling of spring cleaning, purging the closets, getting rid of the unwanted accumulated stuff?

I include noise in this conversation—auditory clutter. Some of us need absolute quiet, while others need soothing or stimulating music to focus best.

Understanding our relationship to the stuff and noise in our environment opens opportunities for self-improvement that don't need to take much time or effort. A little rearranging, taking away some junk, sorting through some piles, and maybe adding some color, pleasing texture, and music. Then we can breathe. We can soothe our overwhelmed senses.

Exercise: Clear Just One Small Space

Ever feel stuck? Can't quite get the project started, or the great idea to emerge? Me too. Here's what I do: clean just one shelf, drawer, or pile (you know what I'm talking about!). Just one. It's small, doable in a short period of time, and not overwhelming. It helps free up just enough energy for you to feel the shift and experience freedom. Be proactive, before the overwhelm and frustration set in. It works every time. And side benefit: if you keep this practice up, you may one day get to a clutter-free home (or workplace).

This practice creates real space for your mind to sink into. It also gives you a place to start, allowing you to initiate and energize forward momentum. You get the promise of follow-through (because it's such a small task) and a sense of completion. It's a small win, but a win all the same. Our spirits thrive on this.

Sleep Neglect

Want to create more space and time in your life for healing? Sleep more. Sleep is the boss. Sleep is our time for renewal and restoration. It's when the toxins are literally swept away from our brains. We all know how toxic it feels not to sleep enough or to have sleep persistently interrupted. And much of this we have control over (moms, dads, and caretakers of babies, you're excused!). We create sleep debt by choosing to stay up late or by powering past our sleepy time with adrenaline, sugar, and stimulants. Or perhaps we spend our evenings taking care of our family's needs instead of our own—you know, making supper, cleaning up, doing laundry, putting the kids to bed—then lay down too exhausted and wired to fall asleep.

If this is you, make sleep your priority, as Mandy did, and take baby steps to make it happen. Then dive into chapter five, RESTORE, for more discussion and action steps for creating beautiful, nourishing, detoxifying, restorative sleep.

ENVIRONMENTAL TOXICITY

The reality is we live in a polluted world. Pollution is driven by countless sources in our increasingly industrialized, fast-paced, efficiency-driven world, including:

- rapid growth of industry that both creates toxins and improperly manages waste products;

- production and widespread use of poisonous pesticides and herbicides;

- the human population explosion, which leads to over-utilization of energy and creation of waste;

- poor management of carbon emissions from automobiles and other fuel-consuming technologies;

- industrialized farming practices that result in over-grazing and nutrient depletion of vast areas of soil;

- extensive deforestation resulting in loss of the earth's natural carbon cleansing potential;

- production of large quantities of toxic, non-biodegradable consumer goods such as plastics;

- simply more people consuming more stuff and using more natural resources—new homes, clothes, on-line retailers direct-to-your-door delivery.

These human practices have come together with enormous, profound, and synergistic effects, resulting not only in the loss of precious natural resources and devastation of our world's natural beauty and diversity, but also in widespread and severe health problems. The epidemics of cancer, obesity, vascular diseases, neurodegenerative disorders, and inflammatory and autoimmune disorders are in large part caused by these toxic influences.

It's a bleak story. Our toxic environment and its negative effects on human health has been so well studied as to be irrefutable at this point, though it is a woefully neglected part of healthcare and social management. Conventional Western medicine does not consider detoxification in its scheme of health considerations. I recently took my American Board of Internal Medicine recertification exam and was horrified that environmental illness and detoxification did not come up even once.

We can't ignore this critical part of our healing. We've got to learn what our enemies are and practice avoidance and protection. What I'm going to tell you about environmental toxicity may feel bleak and depressing, but you need to know the truth.

And know this: there are straightforward action steps we can all make to profoundly reduce the impact of toxicity in our lives.

Pesticides, Herbicides, and Industrial Pollutants

There are literally thousands of chemicals used for eradicating pests and weeds, cleaning, manufacturing processes, and a wide variety of industrial and everyday uses in existence today—and many more are in development. Most of these chemicals are known to cause significant harm to humans and animals. In spite of this they are approved for common usage. They are everywhere, and we can't avoid them completely.

Pesticides are known to be endocrine disrupters and carcinogens. They are linked to infertility, fetal loss, abnormal sexual development, hormone imbalances, autoimmune disorders, and cancers.

Industrial pollutants include a wide variety of chemicals and heavy metals known to cause great harm to all living things. Many of these are difficult to avoid. Developed countries have taken great strides to limit carbon emissions from automobiles and industrial wastes, though developing regions of the world much less so—these pollutants continue to impact us hugely. The EPA has established limitations to industrial pollution and use of harmful chemicals, although the "allowable" levels, while considered "safe" for most people, continue to be harmful and devastating to the most sensitive and vulnerable amongst us.

Glyphosate: Round-Up Is Everywhere

Glyphosate is an herbicide developed by Monsanto that kills weeds in their growing phase. It deserves special attention here because never before in human history has an environmental chemical been used so extensively worldwide and with such carelessness, mostly because we were assured that it was not toxic to human beings. When combined with genetically modified crops resistant to its effects, glyphosate can be used extensively to kill the weeds that would otherwise compete with the crop. This chemical interferes with an enzyme called EPSPS found within plants and bacteria. Blocking this enzyme stops the synthesis of proteins and certain key players in both plant and bacterial metabolism, so growth and survival are not possible.

The prevailing dogma has been that glyphosate is nontoxic to humans because the enzyme EPSPS isn't a part of our physiology. However, this thinking ignores the huge impact of the microbiome (the bacteria that reside within our bodies and play a central role in our physiological function) on human health. It is now known that ingestion of glyphosate causes disruption of our microbiome as well as suppression of important detoxification pathways. It is being linked to numerous human health disorders including neurodegenerative diseases, autism, inflammatory bowel disease, autoimmune disorders and cancer. In March of 2015 the World Health Organization's International Agency for Research on Cancer published a summary of a monograph on glyphosate and classified it as "probably" carcinogenic in humans, based on epidemiological, animal, and in vitro studies.

How to Protect Ourselves from Pesticides, Herbicides, and Industrial Pollutants

There is much we can do to reduce our exposure and protect ourselves from the full impact of environmental pollution:

- Limit our exposure by not bringing toxins into our homes, yards, gardens, and workplaces;

- Use safe and natural ways to address pest and cleaning problems (these can be found through a simple Google inquiry);

- Keep homes and work environments clean, including taking shoes off at the door to prevent tracking in toxins, using air purification systems such as HEPA filters, installing water purification systems, and utilizing the carbon cleaning effects of house plants;

- Bolster our innate mechanisms for processing toxins internally and clear them from the body (We'll address this a bit later in this chapter).

The Ubiquitous Plastics

Plastics are everywhere and in everything. Our water bottles, food containers, plastic wraps, appliances, televisions, and computers. It has been estimated that sixty thousand plastic bags are used by Americans every five seconds. These bags are made from nonrenewable resources. They take huge amounts of energy to manufacture, transport around the world, and recycle. Four percent of the world's oil production is used to make plastic materials, four percent for the energy required in their manufacture, and additional resources for recycling and transportation. Plastics have a colossal impact on our carbon and toxicity footprint.

The pervasive single-use plastic bottles and bags are nonbiodegradable, so they sit in landfills, gradually release toxic chemicals, and litter the entire planet and its oceans. They clog sewage and drainage systems leading to major flooding in developing countries and leach toxic chemicals into the water supplies. They are ingested by or tangled with marine life causing death and deformity. The Great Pacific Garbage Patch, estimated to be twice the size of Hawaii, is a mountain of ocean debris, found in the north Pacific Ocean, caused by plastic bags and other sources of plastics. There are similar garbage patches in the Indian and Atlantic Oceans. These massive accumulations of plastic in our oceans lead to devastation of the surrounding ecology, migrate to distant areas, spread their toxicity, and transport invasive, destructive organic material.

Plastics contain toxic chemicals that we ingest through their use, for example:

- Phthalates: plasticizers found in vinyl flooring and food packaging—most of us have measurable amounts of these carcinogens in our bodies.

- Bisphenol A (BPA): this endocrine disrupter is found in bottles and linings of cans and leeches into our food and drink.

- Polybrominated diphenyl ethers (PBDE's): these are used as flame-retardants added to furniture, mattresses, carpet pads and car seats. These have been associated with thyroid, liver, and neurocognitive disorders.

The process of manufacturing plastics leads to further release of carcinogenic, neurotoxic, and hormone-disruptive chemicals that permeate our entire ecology and persist over long periods of time. Some of the more familiar among these are vinyl chloride (in PVC), dioxins (in PVC), benzene (in polystyrene), phthalates, other plasticizers (in PVC), formaldehyde, and BPA. PVC is particularly dangerous when burned owing to the release of dioxins, which are some of the most harmful of all synthetic compounds. PVC fumes contribute substantially to the toxicity of accidental home or building incinerations.

How to Protect Ourselves from Plastics

We can address this seemingly insurmountable problem with plastic toxicity with very simple, manageable steps to greatly reducing our personal use of plastic materials:

- by being diligent about using non-plastic shopping bags and reusing them,

- by avoiding the purchase and consumption of beverages in plastic containers,

- by not heating food in plastic containers,

- by using reusable non-plastic storage containers,

- and by avoiding use of microplastics in facial and body cleansing products. We can also reduce our consumption of microplastics by using salt sourced from the Himalayas.

Toxic Buildings

Buildings are sources of environmental toxicity that are increasingly recognized as important contributors to human environmental illness.

There are many reasons why our homes, workplaces, and commercial dwellings can become toxic, including:

- chemicals in building materials, furniture, cleaning products, and pesticides;

- poor ventilation and inefficient heating systems that encourage the accumulation of toxins;

- mold toxins, an increasingly acknowledged cause of human illness;

- factors that compound the impact of biological irritants such as crowded work spaces, poor lighting and color, inadequate noise management, prolonged sitting, and long work hours;

- electromagnetic Frequencies (EMF) created by electrical systems, electronics, and wireless networks that may be harmful to sensitive people.

Toxic and Irritating Food

Many commonly consumed foods rank right up there with the worst environmental toxins. Our food supply is now filled with what my mentor, and visionary founder of Functional Medicine, Dr. Jeffrey Bland, refers to as "new to nature molecules." In addition to pharmaceuticals, these include manmade synthetic and altered foods and food additives designed to make food more resistant to spoilage, easier to package, more colorful, more convenient, and generally more pleasing to the consumer. The processing of food in these ways strips it of nutrient value and adds toxicity, leading directly to changes in biology and genetic expression that make people ill.

Most processed foods have undergone alterations in their basic structures to make them more stable or amenable to combination with other ingredients. This process leads inevitably to loss of nutrients and enhanced exposure to the damaging effects of oxidation and spoilage. In the food industry this necessitates the addition of preservatives and "fortification" with vitamins. In the end we have something that is less than real, less fresh, and far inferior to what we can prepare in our own kitchens. Rule of thumb: eat only real, unprocessed, fresh food for highest nutrient value, taste, and safety.

Another noteworthy category of toxic food is sugar. Sugar, including the simple sugars found in cane, honey, maple syrup, and other plant syrups, is not an essential human nutrient, and with regular or excessive ingestion acts as a toxin. Sugar consumption in excess is as toxic as any environmental chemical exposure due to its dangerous biological effects. In fact, sugar has become the most ubiquitous and harmful toxin known to mankind due to its abundance and massive consumption by people worldwide. We're all familiar with the disastrous consequences—an epidemic of obesity, diabetes, inflammatory vascular disease, cancers, and more—directly related to excess ingestion of sugar in its various forms.

Many other foods make us sick and toxic. It is now recognized that there are innumerable ways we can become chemically and immunologically sensitive to proteins and other constituents of foods. These reactions directly trigger inflammatory and biochemical havoc that make us sick. The details of these reactions are explored in chapter seven, Nourish.

The Foundational Intensive Nutrition Energy (FINE) and Gut-Immune Restoration Intensive Nutrition (GRIN) food plans are examples of eating strategies that remove the problematic irritant foods while providing nutrient density to support our biology. These will be reviewed in detail in chapter seven.

LETTING GO OF TOXICITY—FINDING OUT WHERE YOU MIGHT BE STUCK

Now that we have examined the different kinds of toxicity we experience in our lives, it's time to work on recognizing which ones are most threatening to our own individual healing. We can't live in a bubble—we're all part of the big web of life. But we can take control. There is much we can let go of to make space for healing.

Quiz: Life Toxicity Inventory—Where You Might Be Stuck

Answer the following questions with a "yes" or "no." Give yourself one point for each "yes" and zero points for each "no."

Tally your overall score as well as scores for each section. These serve only the purpose of showing you what parts of the Let Go domain deserve your attention. The higher your score, the more chance there is that toxicity is a significant player in the current state of your health and wellbeing.

Guilt, Shame, and Judgment

- Do you blame yourself for not feeling well or your best?

- Do you feel like a failure for attempts to heal that have not worked out?

- Do you feel guilt or shame for low energy, lack of motivation, or illness?

- Do you feel that if you could only "get it right" you'd feel better?

- Are you hard on yourself about self-care?

- Do you feel like you're never enough just as you are?

Old Ways and Habits

- Are there regular parts of your daily routine that you know aren't good for you, but you do them anyway?

- Are there parts of your regular daily routine that you would like to change?

- Do you skimp on relaxation?

- Do you wish there were more play, laughter, and fun in your daily life?

- Do you eat food that you sense is not good for you?

- Do you eat too much?

- Do you drink less than two quarts of water (sixty-four ounces) per day?

- Do you spend a significant part of your day sitting?

- Do you burn the candle at both ends and consistently feel time pressured?

- Do you have trouble implementing new healthy activities in your daily routine?

Negative Energy of People

- Do you feel anxious or overwhelmed around certain people in your life?

- Are there people in your life who don't support you or your dreams and desires?

- Are there people in your life who are critical of you?

- Do you avoid crowds?

- Do you sometimes say "yes," to people, when you really mean "no?"

- Do you tend to defer to the desires and demands of others rather than your own?

Distraction

- Do you drive while talking on your cell phone (even hands-free)?

- Do you talk on the phone while out walking or shopping?

- Do you have a hard time disengaging from social media?

- Do you watch or read the news daily?

- Do you have a hard time pulling yourself away from news notifications?

- Do you watch TV for more than an hour every day?

- Do you have cluttered surfaces or drawers in your house or workplace?

- Do you ever lose track of things among the clutter?

- Do you ever feel anxious or overwhelmed by clutter in your living or work environment?

Not Enough Sleep or Rest

- Do you habitually skimp on sleep, knowing you need more?

- Do you forego sleeping enough to stay up for other things?

- Do you not sleep well—either struggle to fall asleep or wake up during the night?

- Do you wake up in the morning feeling tired or unrestored?

- Do you consistently get fewer than eight hours of sleep per night?

- Do you do everything fast and rushed to cram it all into your day?

Environmental Pollution

- Are you exposed to pesticides or industrial pollutants?

- Do you use plastic containers for heating or storing food?

- Do you use single-use plastic water bottles?

- Do you have a wireless network in your home that is on 24/7?

- Do you sleep with a cell phone turned on in your bedroom?

- Do you live or work in a poorly ventilated building?

HEAL KARYN SHANKS MD

- Do you live on or near a farm that uses pesticides and herbicides?

- Do you eat nonorganic produce, meat, or animal milk products?

Toxic and Irritating Food

- Do you eat sugar of any kind (table sugar, fructose, agave, honey, maple syrup, and so on)?

- Do you eat grains (even "healthy" whole grains)?

- Do you have a hard time staying away from sugar?

- Do you eat/drink food containing high fructose corn syrup?

- Do you eat any foods that make you feel bad?

- Do you feel like you drink too much alcohol?

- Do you ever feel sluggish, bloated, or unwell after a meal?

- Do you have irritable bowel syndrome (IBS) or small intestinal bacterial overgrowth (SIBO)?

Stress

- Do you often feel stressed-out or overwhelmed?

- Do you do everything quickly and rushed to cram it all into your day?

- Do you feel like you consistently fail to meet your expectations for yourself or for the day?

- Do you consistently leave little time for your own rest, relaxation, fun, or restoration?

LET GO!

Acknowledge Where You're Stuck and Own It

Accept responsibility for the fact that you (yes, you!) have toxic habits (we all do!). Then give them a name—you know them. What are your old ways and habits that no longer serve you?

Take Baby Steps

Change the small things first or small parts of the big things. It's okay if it doesn't all get done today—*it can't*. Less is always more. Make sure your actions are doable and sustainable. Chewing off too much leads to failure and frustration. Small steps lead to small wins and that feels good to the soul and creates a foundation to build upon.

Create Time

Yes, you *do* have time. Realize that. Acknowledge that. Your current priorities may not support what you want. Your call is to slow down and let go of the distractions and time wasters that get in your way.

Make a List

Make a list of the old ways and habits that you know make you feel sick, depleted, or overwhelmed. Include any of the "yes" responses from your Life Toxicity Inventory. Write them all down. Do this quickly and don't limit yourself—just blurt them all out. Realize that you don't have to change all of them today, but this exercise helps us get the ball rolling and gives us a focus for beginning this journey.

Then, Choose Three Small Things

Pick three small things from your list—or take a big thing and break it down into three smaller pieces. Write down how you plan to change or let go of these starting today.

Stick with three—three is a power theme for human engagement—compelling the mind, enhancing memory and pleasure, and increasing chances for success. And keep them small. Start today.

Always Give Yourself Thanks

Now, congratulate yourself! You're building on the healing already begun, opening more space, letting go, and making room for healing. Getting better and stronger already! And you did this all for yourself.

HOW TO LET GO OF BIOLOGICAL TOXICITY

Bolster Your Body's Innate Detoxification Systems

So far, we've talked about trying to avoid and eliminate the many life toxins that get in the way of our healing and letting go of bad habits and old stories that get us stuck. But in spite of our best efforts, some toxins will get in. This is especially true for environmental toxins. That's the world we live in. But we're not helpless. Not only can we take responsibility for avoiding them in the ways already discussed, we can also bolster our bodies' innate capacity to remove toxins.

What is "Detoxification"?

Detoxification is a core physiologic process of our bodies, designed to manage the toxins we are exposed to from both our internal and external sources. It operates continuously and demands a constant supply of energy and essential nutrients to function optimally.

Detoxification is not something we can sustain with a twice yearly seven-day "detox" program, or occasional cleanse, colonic, or sauna. It's a 24/7 proposition, and to work well for us, it must be supported daily.

Detoxification is part of the innate intelligence of our bodies yet can become overwhelmed by toxin exposure when there are inadequate nutrients or energy to manage it. When this happens, the toxins have an opportunity to interfere with our bodies' complex physiology, making us more vulnerable to damage, disease, and dysfunction. Detoxification problems are important players in our most common health problems.

How to Achieve Optimal Detoxification—The Basics

To stay safe and healthy, we must support the path toxins take from point of entry into the body all the way to exit. This is detoxification, a resource- and energy-expensive process that prepares toxins for elimination and supports the channels through which they must pass. Toxins must be made water-soluble by the liver for transport through blood, bile, urine, sweat, and exhaled moisture. The flow of toxins through their respective fluids, and the function of their exit pathways (gut, kidneys, sweat) must be supported and maintained.

Avoid Environmental Toxins

Take precautions to avoid the environmental pollutants, pesticides, plastics, toxic internal environments, and toxic and irritating food as discussed in the previous section on environmental toxicity.

Eat Nutrient-Dense Food to Support Detoxification

The standard American diet (SAD) is nutrient poor and contains many food irritants. This combination leads to blocks in detoxification because there simply are not enough resources for this energy- and nutrient-expensive process to proceed. The SAD's impact on detoxification and health is compounded by common medication use that causes damage to our primary detoxification organs—the liver, gut, and kidneys—or overwhelm their capacity to keep up with toxin clearing.

The intensive nutrition required to run the operation of detoxification is described in the chapter seven. While we are all genetically unique, and our nutritional requirements for optimal detoxification will differ, the food plans described in chapter seven will provide templates that will meet the needs of most. A well-trained Functional Medicine practitioner will be able to help those of you with additional needs.

Stay Well Hydrated

Water assists in the transport of toxins from all sites within the body to the point of elimination. Most people require a minimum of two to three quarts of water daily.

Encourage Good Bile Flow

This will be accomplished by including healthy fat with each meal and snack. Bile is released with the ingestion of fat, serving as a fat emulsifier, allowing it to be absorbed through the gut lining. This regular release of bile allows for the toxins, transformed in the liver, to be released frequently and eventually eliminated from the body via the intestinal tract.

Keep Bowels Healthy and Moving

Regular and complete daily bowel movements are essential for proper elimination of toxins that have been processed in the liver, dumped into the bile, and released into the intestines. Adequate water intake, movement, dietary fiber, and a healthy microbiome are essential.

By following the primarily plant-based food plans in chapter seven, and by taking a good quality, multi-species probiotic daily, most people will enjoy healthy bowel elimination. For those who are not able to easily move their bowels in large quantity on a daily basis, it is important to work with a Functional Medicine specialist to help you with this. Additional fiber, magnesium, or mild intestinal stimulants may be needed.

Consume Detoxification Support Nutrition Daily

It is important to consume food rich in nutrition to support all aspects of detoxification and energy production. You'll find this foundational support in the FINE and GRIN food plans in chapter seven. Consider using supplemental nutrition to support detoxification.[5]

Sweat, Move, Exercise, Breathe Deeply, Sleep Well

These are all key aspects of maintaining healthy flow of toxins out of our bodies. Sweat is one of the major routes we use for toxin elimination, in addition to the gut, kidneys, and lungs. Any movement or activity that elevates the core temperature of the body sufficiently to induce a profuse sweat is all you need. This may include intense exercise, a hot bath or shower, being outside on a hot day, or use of a sauna designed to raise core body temperature. Far-infrared saunas are your best bet and there are many small, affordable versions available to purchase for personal use. We'll explore movement and sleep in depth in upcoming chapters.

LAST THOUGHTS

Now we've created space—sacred space for *us*. For who we are, our healing, our potential. We've identified the old, the worn-out, the toxic—the obstacles to our healing. And we've nourished our minds and bodies with strategies for letting that all go.

Now, we call in the love! The first nutrient of our healing. To fertilize the terrain of our hearts, minds, and bodies for what's to come. Onward to our next domain: LOVE—Love and Connect (Yourself First, Then Others).

----

[5] See *A Detoxification Primer: How to Let Go of Biological Toxicity*: karynshanksmd.com/2018/12/09/a-detoxification-primer/

Chapter Three

LOVE

Love and Connect
(Yourself First, Then Others)

We created space within ourselves for healing by letting go—we had to show up, go slow, and pay attention. We're prepared now to open space within our deserving hearts. To welcome love—love that mirrors our true nature (have you forgotten?). We allow that love to expand and elevate us.

We learn to love ourselves through our thoughts and actions first—becoming strong and whole. Then extend our big blazing hearts out to others—creating the circle of love that is the strength of our humanity and the source of our healing.

LOVE IS US

Love. This is it. This is *us*. This is why we're here. Love is who we are and all that we aspire to. Our healing, our energy, our lives are all about love. Love is our destination, our purpose, and our path. When we're in the flow with love, we thrive. But although love is all around us, we can lose our connection to it. This is our work in this chapter—to create space for love.

But, first, how do we define love? The word, itself, is a container for so many varied and nuanced notions about what love means. And there are so many kinds of love: love of family, love of our children, romantic or sexual love, love of our communities, love of art.

For the purpose of our discussion, I'm going to work with love not as a singularly definable term, but rather as an idea to represent the energy that is exchanged between us and others that is pleasurable, elevating, and binds us together. I'm also going to speak of love as a verb. Love takes on more value when it supports, connects, inspires, and empowers.

LOVE HEALS

Love is powerful stuff.

Ever notice how someone's simple act or words of kindness can completely transform how you feel? Perhaps shifting you out of a dark mood? Changing the course of your whole day—or even your whole life?

That's the healing power of love. Love is physical and emotional energy that transcends time and space. Love is a catapult, a healing balm, a magical and mysterious connection that exists among us. It connects us with one another, our children, animals, nature, and the world around us. It moves heaven and earth, with the power to transform our greatest suffering into redemption and recovery. It softens and lightens us, lifting life's burdens, while shining light on the beauty all around us.

Love can be the simple things. The smile of a passing stranger. The encouragement from a friend. The many courtesies, welcomings, friendliness, inclusions, generosities, touch, and kindnesses that we receive—and give—in so many ways. They all count. They all make us rise. They all touch and restore us. In all of its nuanced ways, love heals us.

Love-Heals Science: HeartMath

Modern science is showing that love is not just the nebulous, touchy-feely add-on to our physical lives. On the contrary, research from the HeartMath Institute reveals love's power to heal and the innate intelligence of the heart. Their work shows that love is an inseparable, real, and necessary part of our physical and emotional health. Through its exquisite physical circuitry, love not only makes us feel better, it leads to physiological changes that strengthen and heal.

HeartMath researchers have observed that approximately seventy percent of all information shared between the heart and brain moves from the heart *to* the brain. The heart—our circulatory hub and physical center for love—is also a key neurological control center with powerful connections to the brain. The heart influences how we think, feel, make decisions, and remember.

Further, they've shown that love, the emotion we most commonly attribute to the heart, actually makes the heart perform better. The healthiest hearts possess high "heart rate variability" (HRV), a measure of the heart's adaptability to life's challenges. A healthy heart is able to adapt well to moment by moment physiological changes by varying its rate of contraction—its HRV—managing blood flow in response to the changing demands placed upon it. A heart with low HRV cannot adapt quickly and represents a body that has lost resilience. Researchers have found that low HRV is associated with a large range of health problems, including heart disease, fetal distress, autonomic nervous system dysfunction, asthma, anxiety, depression, and diabetes.

Loving thoughts and emotions increase HRV and are linked to improvements in a wide array of health attributes. The HeartMath folks came up with an extraordinarily simple exercise to help people actively optimize HRV—so simple that anyone can do it. Subjects are prompted to bring to mind memories of loving thoughts and experiences, engendering loving emotions within the chest, or "heart space." Subjects might think of something or someone they love while touching the center of their chest to conjure the sensation of love. Using a handheld biofeedback device that measures HRV, researchers have observed how HRV improves with this exercise. With regular practice, numerous positive health outcomes are created: healthier stress responses, improved mood and cognitive function, lower risk of heart attack, less anxiety, and improved asthma, to name just a few.

In addition, HeartMath research shows that negative emotions, such as anger and frustration, decrease HRV. When persistent, such negative emotions are strongly associated with adverse health conditions, including heart attack, stroke, and suicide.

Practice: Feel the Love—A Heart-Centered Meditation

Sit quietly. Close your eyes. Breathe in and out deeply and slowly. Let go of all of your current worries and concerns (they will wait for you, trust me). Place your hands over your heart, right in the center of your chest. Breathe in deeply there. Focus your breath in the center of your chest. Let the breath expand there, then let it all out. Let it go.

Now, think about something or someone who you completely love. Who pops into your mind? A child? Pet? Friend? Spouse? Whomever or whatever it is, think about them. Let that feeling of love fill your heart. Let it wash over you.

What physical sensations or emotions did you feel?

That's you. Love is in you.

Enjoy this simple sensation. And if you didn't connect to it this time, not to worry—we all vary greatly in our abilities to feel and observe what's happening on the inside. Connecting to love may take practice. You might have competing thoughts getting in the way right now. Come back and try this again later.

Consider how simple that exercise was. A few simple breaths and a single thought or memory, and the energy of love touched, moved, or possibly exploded within your heart. The emotion and energy of love resides right there within your body. And you can conjure it up at any moment with just a simple intention and memory of a loving presence in your life. This is one powerful way to practice love and to experience the ease with which it can flow into your body. As the HeartMath researchers have shown us, love practice de-stresses us, increases our mind power, and makes us healthier.

The Healing Power of Love and Intimacy

We're all familiar with the research that shows married people live longer than unmarried people. More recently, we've learned this observation applies to all partnered people. In fact, when combining the results for married and unmarried-but-cohabiting partners, the survival effects of partnership compared to married only are strengthened.[6] Of course, this applies primarily to *happily* married and partnered people. They enjoy greater happiness, longer lives, and fewer health problems. Unhappily married and partnered people, on the other hand, have higher blood pressure, more stress, and a greater number of health problems.

The scientific literature is full of evidence about the health benefits of being in loving intimate relationships: lower blood pressure, less depression, faster wound healing, enhanced immune function with fewer colds and acute illnesses, lower stress levels, and less anxiety.

Why is this? Well, love is physical. It has a biology. It changes our brains and manifests biochemical changes in our bodies that lead to lower stress, greater happiness, and increased survival. It's just plain good for us.

Even physical expressions of love are healing. Hugging and hand holding increases our levels of the bonding hormone, oxytocin. This leads to less stress, lower blood pressure, elevated mood, and increased tolerance for pain. Kissing has been shown to reduce stress and cholesterol levels and increase relationship satisfaction. And sex, well, it's the elixir of vibrant health and happiness, boasting enhanced immunity with fewer sick days, increased libido, better bladder control in women, lower blood pressure, lower risk for heart attack, less pain, lowered risk for prostate cancer in men, improved sleep, lower stress levels, and it counts as exercise!

The authenticity and intimacy we bring to our relationships is also key. As Brené Brown, in her famous work on vulnerability[7] has shown, risking vulnerability and whole-heartedness within our relationships makes us feel happier and able to connect with one another more deeply. Even within the broader context of social relationships—strong

---

[6] Sebastian Franke and Hill Kulu. *Cause-specific mortality by partnership status: simultaneous analysis using longitudinal data from England and Wales.* J Epi Comm Health, BMJ. 2018; 72(9): dx.doi.org/10.1136/jech-2017-210339.

[7] Brené Brown. *Rising Strong.* 2015.

connections to friends, family, neighbors, and colleagues—the willingness to be vulnerable and authentic has been shown to increase survival by fifty percent.

LOVE IS WISDOM

"A loving heart is the truest wisdom."

—*Charles Dickens*

The great masters and teachers of this world have long told us that love matters most, love heals all, we must always follow our hearts, and our hearts are the seats of the greatest wisdom.

None of us are strangers to the wisdom of love. Don't our hearts always tell us who and what's good for us, what contains the answers we seek, or what we most need? And don't we always regret it when we fail to heed what our hearts have to tell us?

We call this heart wisdom many things: inner wisdom, the small quiet voice, intuition, inner knowing, or the heartbeat of God. It's the truth of what we know—*truly know*—deep within our heart of hearts. It's a knowing that is innate to all of us and guides us effortlessly once we learn to recognize it, take time for it, listen to it, and trust it.

This wisdom of the heart—love, Universal love, the love of God or nature, whatever you conceive it to be—is accessible to all of us. We're all born with it. But it's tricky. It gets mixed up in the noise of our busy minds, our saturated senses, our stories, and the thoughts, advice, and dictums of others. How do we learn to recognize it?

Love is like our own internal GPS system, revealing our terrain, and guiding us on our true path. If we listen, and trust it, we always seem to find our way.

We also all know what happens when we ignore our heart's guidance. We get off track. We make mistakes we shouldn't make. We blurt out hurtful things we regret.

My Heart's Wisdom Solved a Riddle

A long time ago I was wrestling with uncomfortable feelings about a friend who seemed competitive and jealous of my accomplishments. I found myself avoiding her, angry and, of course, guilty for how I felt.

One day, while out on a long walk, stewing in my juices over it, quite suddenly and unexpectedly, a voice rose up from my heart, quiet and soft. It said, "Karyn, she's just trying to prove herself to you." It was kind, loving, and forgiving to us both, and answered the puzzle. I knew it to be the wisdom of my heart. It helped me see the situation with new clarity. I was able to talk to my friend and work things out.

My heart cut right through the stories circling through my head. We all do this—our stories come at us as "the truth," "the way it is," or "how I understand it to be." We often forget that "the truth" is really *our* truth. My "jealous" and "competitive" friend was really just wrestling with her own feelings of unworthiness and seeking my approval.

My first clue that I was dealing with a story I'd created to explain my friend's behavior, was that I was conflicted, angry, and didn't know how to handle the situation. The quiet, soft voice of my heart cut through the confusion and told the truth. I felt absolutely clear.

How to Recognize Heart Wisdom

I think it's helpful to look for the warning signs that tell us when we're dealing with stories we've created to explain our circumstances, and not the clear, pure guidance of our heart's wisdom. If the voice is judging (telling you "good" or "bad," "right" or "wrong"), condemning ("what an idiot!"), or disempowering to you or anyone else, it is NEVER true wisdom from the heart. Not ever. Those are always stories.

Does the inner voice preface its advice with "you should" or "it would be best" or "you must"? These preambles usually represent the dictums of someone else, or a societal norm, not your own inner guidance. Always question these. Don't trust them to be your own true inner wisdom.

If the inner voice you hear makes you feel guilt or shame, it is not wisdom. It is not a voice from the heart. It's a toxic voice and you should send it packing.

How about the fearful voice? When should you heed this wisdom? On the one hand, fear is helpful and vital. Our brains were designed to keep us alive by keeping us out of harm's way. Fear is the innate emotional tool our brains use to get our attention, lead us to quick action, and remove us from danger. Jumping away from the oncoming car or avoiding a toxic person who means us harm are critical to our survival. But when is fear about true danger, rather than our *assumptions* about what will happen if we make a choice, take a risk, or accept personal responsibility?

Pay attention to fear. Then, look for the "shoulds" and "should nots," the guilt and shame. Risk taking, uncertainty, and vulnerability are scary but they're never judging or disempowering. The worst-case scenario is always a story[8]—never wisdom of the heart.

True inner wisdom is always the voice of love. It may bring a warning or ask for correction of our behavior, but it does so in a nonjudging and loving way. Our heart's true wisdom will never bring information about you or others that is not based in love.

Practice: A Love Is Wisdom Exercise

Let's take a moment to tap into your heart's wisdom.

Consider a problem or question you need clear guidance about. Ask for help out loud (or write it down on a piece of paper—or the margin of this book) and express your intention to listen. Place your hands over your heart. Breathe deeply in and out here, right into your heart. Feel the sensations that arise (or don't arise) in your body as you pose your question. How does it feel? Warm? Positive? Does it feel like a "yes"? Or, is it negative, cold, restricted, a pulling away, a "no"? Are there any words that come forth? Do tears come to your eyes?

The heart's wisdom can hit us between the eyes, or it can be very subtle. Recognizing it takes practice, patience, and careful intentional listening. We may put out the questions but not have answers come right away. We might be distracted and not hear or feel the subtle ways the answers present themselves. Or perhaps our guidance is to keep chewing

---

[8] We'll explore and work more with the stories of our lives in chapter eight, DISCOVER.

on the question—it's just not ready yet. Be patient. Keep asking. And live the questions. The answers will come.

LOVE IS SOCIAL CONNECTION

We were born to be social creatures. We're at our healthiest when living in meaningful community with others—belonging to our families and friends, connected to our communities and tribes. Knowing we are essential parts of something larger than ourselves makes us strong, helps us feel safe.

Social connection protects our health. Studies show that when we perceive our social connection as high, we live longer, enjoy more robust immunity with lower rates of infection and cancer. We experience less depression and anxiety, have higher self-esteem, empathy, and more stable emotions.

Believing that we are disconnected from others is more dangerous than smoking, high blood pressure, or obesity. Studies on persistent loneliness show higher levels of inflammation, more anxiety and depression, slower recovery from disease and injury, increased antisocial behavior and violence, and increased risk of suicide. Our brains interpret loneliness and social isolation as profound dangers and threats to our very survival, and they defensively place our stress systems on high alert. This leads to elevated stress hormone levels and massive changes in our physiology, gene expression, and behavior to support the body's response to conditions that have the potential to kill us. There is an observed forty to sixty-four percent increased risk for dementia in those who feel lonely.[9] It is now understood that beta-amyloid and other toxic proteins deposited in

---

Angela R. Sutin, et al. *Loneliness and Risk of Dementia.* 26 October 2018. J Gerontology: Series B, gby112: doi.org/10.1093/geronb/gby112.

the brains of Alzheimer's patients, as well as those with other forms of dementia, are stress molecules produced by the immune system in response to such threats to our survival—the unremitting stress of loneliness and social isolation.

Introverts need not worry, though, as the benefits of social connection do not depend on the number of friends we have. What support us are our perceptions about the quality of our connections and the sense of belonging we establish through our nuanced participation in our communities and the people in our lives.

Roseto, Pennsylvania—How Social Connection Overrides Unhealthy Habits

A small community of Italian Americans from Roseto, Pennsylvania became famous for their unusually excellent health characteristics in spite of potentially dangerous daily health habits. These immigrants, shunned by the haughty English and Welsh who dominated the region in the early 1900s, formed their own tight knit community out of necessity. They ran their own businesses, attended their own churches, and collaborated for all community services. Every household was comprised of at least three generations.

The Roseto folks labored hard, smoked, consumed alcohol heavily, and ate food high in unhealthy fats, leaving behind the plant and healthy fat-based Mediterranean diets of their ancestors for economic reasons. In spite of these normally detrimental lifestyle characteristics the Roseto community was observed to have only half the risk of developing heart disease compared to all other communities in the United States.

In time the Roseto community prospered. It was the first generation's aspiration that their children would become educated and not have to work as hard as they did. The young ones went off to college, a luxury the earlier generations did not have. Many of this younger generation left the community behind—along with its traditions and close

---

Tjalling Jan Holwerda, et al. *Feelings of loneliness, but not social isolation, predict dementia onset: results from the Amsterdam Study of the Elderly (AMSTEL)*. 2013, Volume 85, issue 2: dx.doi.org/10.1136/jnnp-2012-302755.

HEAL KARYN SHANKS MD

interdependence—for a "better life." That new independence came with a price: eventually, the rate of heart attacks among the younger generation reverted to the national norm.

One hypothesis is that what impacted this community's health so profoundly were their close relationships and strong social support, providing the community members with a powerful sense of security and belonging. This strong community connection ameliorated the stress of suboptimal diets, smoking, and harsh working conditions, protecting them from the physiological changes that lead to disease. This has been dubbed the "Roseto effect," and it has become synonymous with love in action—how community and close connection to others is good medicine.

FIRST, WE LOVE OURSELVES

This love we speak of that is us, that is the foundation of our healing, has to start with us. Self-love is the nourishment we must have to jumpstart and sustain our healing and to reach out all around us to create and inspire love in all of our relationships.

Love. It's big. It's grand and glorious. In fact, it can be so big and grand and glorious that it can be frightening, confusing, and overwhelming. We know it's the essence of who we are as people and the ultimate core to our healing, but it can get lost—or rather, we lose sight of it. Not only in the muck and fatigue of life, but also in the busy-ness and constant to-do-ing of life. How do we bring it into our complicated lives? Well, as always, we start with ourselves.

Sally's Story: The Weight of the World

Sally was a client of mine who skidded into extreme exhaustion after the birth of her second child. She went back to her full-time job after a six-week maternity leave and found herself working eight-hour days, picking up her three-year-old daughter and new baby at daycare on the way home, fixing supper, putting the kids to bed, then doing all of the household chores before collapsing into bed herself. It didn't occur to her to ask her husband for help. He was the major breadwinner for the family, after all. Sally was the living embodiment of the idea that a "good" wife bears all, does it all, and puts her needs last.

I first saw her about a year into this saga when she was barely making it. Her sleep was short and not of good quality. She often had a hard time falling asleep and would be awakened by one or both children multiple times through the night. She woke up in the mornings feeling exhausted, stunned by her alarm going off far earlier than she was ready for. She had migraine headaches, vague joint pain, constipation, dry skin, weight gain around the middle, sugar cravings, and depression. She felt trapped.

She had become completely overwhelmed and was on the brink of emotional disaster. She was sick. This life was not sustainable.

This is where Sally's work had to begin: with self-love. Intellectually she got it, but in practice she still believed that it was solely up to her to take care of her family, work—the world. *This was her story*. She was so physically depleted and lacking in energy that she didn't have the emotional fire to advocate for herself, to ask for help, or to set personal boundaries. She was tanked.

I had her start with a few very simple steps that she felt she could manage. We negotiated these carefully because the balance of her life was precarious. While sitting in my office, she crafted simple affirmations about honoring herself. On note cards she wrote: "I honor myself," "I am worthy of my time and attention," "I receive the love and support that I need," "I am fully supported by the Divine Universe." She planned to copy these onto sticky notes and place them on her bathroom mirror, in the kitchen, and on her desk at work—places where she would see them often and sink herself into them. As she wrote and said these affirmations out loud, she told me she felt a palpable release. She felt the space they created for something new—something for *her*.

She also agreed to very small healthy changes in her food plan, sleep schedule, and movement to get her feeling better faster. But baby steps, so she could succeed at them and not pile on guilt about not following them. She planned to avoid sugar and add more vegetables to her diet. She moved up her bedtime by just half an hour, and she enlisted her husband's help with the nightly chores. I suggested she stand more at work, use the stairs instead of the elevator, take a bag and carry groceries at the store rather than use a cart, and take short walks with the kids on weekends. She immediately had a standing desk installed in her office.

She gradually made progress. The positive affirmations had a powerful effect on her, bringing relief, inspiring new hope, and reinforcing what she already knew—that it was not just okay but necessary to tend to herself and her needs first. And instead of the backlash and disappointment from her family she expected, they supported her. Her husband was happy to help out, and everyone has benefitted from her more relaxed and lighthearted presence. She continues to be a work in progress but has made huge strides and is feeling much better.

Dare to Receive Love

> *"Your task is not to seek for love, but merely to seek and find all the barriers within yourself that you have built against it."*

—*Rumi*

Many of us are adept at giving to others but have difficulty with receiving. Perhaps it's in our training. Our culture teaches us that it is better to give than to receive. This is especially true for women who, even to this day, are taught the virtues of caretaking. We do it well. We have learned well from our mothers and grandmothers how to work and raise the kids and clean the house and fix the meals. Not that there is anything inherently wrong with any of these things. It's just that we get so immersed in giving that we forget to ask for help (or feel guilty about doing so). But what *is* asking for help? It's opening ourselves to receive care from someone else—to receiving love.

My Story

My early years were spent growing up in a very stressed household. My young parents had four children by their early twenties and found their way in life without much outside support. That was what you did in the late 1950s. They did well in many ways: my dad completed college and went to work, eventually starting his own architecture firm. My mom managed our complex household on a strict budget and took care of us kids, which in those days meant making most of our clothes and cooking food from scratch.

I think they did an amazing job under the circumstances. There were many good times, and I have wonderful childhood memories, yet there was also a lot of anxiety and anger that would spill out unexpectedly. This left a vivid and profound impression on me. I quietly took it all in and made sense of it in the way only a highly sensitive, introverted, and intuitive child could. I learned to protect myself. I learned the virtues of being quiet and stoic. And since the stress in my environment was always about me (at least according to my young survival-oriented brain) I learned that everything needed to be just right, just so, perfect.

Fast forward decades. My fierce independence, strong work ethic, unrelenting tenacity, and drive to always do more and better made me successful in many ways. But my level of vigilance was not sustainable. My health suffered and I distanced myself from the people who wanted to get closer. I thought my stoicism was strength and my perfectionism about striving to be the best that I could be, but I was wrong. It was fear. I did not trust others with the real me and I was relentlessly pursuing an ideal that simply wasn't possible.

As I described in the introduction to this book, I hit a crisis point of severe fatigue and troublesome symptoms in my mid-thirties. I had to reach out for help, but this was something I did not know how to do. It was terrifying. And yet as I did, people stepped up for me. People took care of me, mentored and guided me, and eventually helped me heal. I had to learn to open my heart and face my vulnerability about exposing my true self. And when I did the love came in. To my surprise people liked me—imperfections and all. In fact, they liked me more. They valued the me I had tried to hide. I encounter the very same thing in many of my clients. A critical part of our healing is learning to ask for and receive love.

This part of our recovery is as vital as good food, sleep, movement, meditation, and the many practices and therapies that support us. It's what heals us all. Love heals.

Self-Love is Our True Nature and the Foundation of All Healing

"Love yourself first and everything else falls into line. You really have to love yourself to get anything done in this world."

—Lucille Ball

This is where the rubber meets the road. To create the time, space, and energy for the self-care that leads to healing, we must love ourselves first and make ourselves our top priority. Self-love energizes and prioritizes the self-care that leads to our energy, potential, and healing.

We're wired for love in countless ways—but we often leave ourselves out of the equation. As we saw with Sally, self-love gets buried by duty to others first. It gets lost in fear and worry, stress and overwork, unworthiness and loneliness. It's cast aside under the muck of negative life experiences and false stories we've been told.

This is our lesson: we intrinsically deserve—and *require*—our own attention, compassion, and care. Our healing can't go on without it. *We* can't go on without it.

Self-Love Is Not Selfish

Putting self-love first strengthens us for others. It's not selfish. We must care for ourselves before we can make the most effective and valuable contributions to others.

This isn't fluffy positive thinking. This is the way our personal and social relationships operate best. There's a reason the airlines always tell us to secure our own oxygen mask before helping those around us. If we don't put our own mask on first when the cabin pressure is compromised, our oxygen-deprived brains won't get it together well enough to be of useful assistance to those around us. The same principle applies to every other aspect of our lives. When we love and care for ourselves first, we're better, stronger, and more competent for others. When we don't, we're deprived of exactly what we need in order to succeed.

One of the most common problems I hear about in my consultation room is how clients don't make themselves a priority. Most bad habits—not eating well, not sleeping enough, not exercising, not playing or having fun, and so on—stem from people not leaving room for themselves in their own lives. They fill their days with obligations to everyone else and leave themselves out. Coming in last means illness, dysfunction, and misery.

And how does a life of self-neglect play out, ultimately, for family, friends, and coworkers? That exhaustion, suffering, and incapacitation impacts everyone. When we suffer, everyone suffers with us.

Practice: Wait! You're Not a Lost Cause!

Let's take a break for a moment from berating ourselves for not loving ourselves enough or not putting ourselves into enough of a priority position in our lives. That all will come as we practice. While it's true, so many of us don't love ourselves enough, we're probably not starting from scratch! Most of us do honor ourselves through our actions and intentions every day, even if we don't carry this practice into all parts of our lives. Self-love is innate—we're born with it. Just look at the way small children celebrate themselves and stake claim to what they need from others. Let's pause for a brief reflective exercise to remind us of our own ability to honor ourselves.

First, think about something nice you do for yourself daily, no matter how small you think it is. Perhaps you make a nice cup of coffee or tea for yourself, enjoy a long hot shower, leisurely read the paper, take time to eat lunch, talk to a friend, go for a walk, or pet your dog.

When you've recalled a few such things, be there for a moment, and remember—see, hear, taste, smell, touch—the details. Most importantly, remember how they made you feel.

Now consider: How do these habits or practices make you feel? Important? Relaxed? Rewarded? Consoled? Uplifted? Peaceful?

Then: Carry that feeling with you into other parts of your life. This is you. This is how you should feel—loved, nourished, and supported—always and in all things.

Know that you are intrinsically wired for self-love and express it daily in some small way or another. This practice can be expanded into all aspects of your life.[10]

Self-Love is a *Verb!*

Self-love is what we *do* for ourselves. It's not just a nice feel-good platitude—it must be fueled by action to transform our lives and the lives of those we love. Although it may sound counterintuitive, we don't have to *feel* it to create it and have it work for us. That spontaneous feeling of joyful love and acceptance of ourselves can be hard—especially when we're suffering, tired, or overwhelmed. The buoyant kind of love comes with practice.

You Are Worthy

Be certain of this: if you feel unworthy or unlovable, *you are ... well, wrong!*

Your greatest, truest, most beautiful being is absolutely inside you and has been there all along just waiting for you to wake up to it. This beautiful you must have your full attention and acknowledgment to come forth and shine its light into the world.

This will be your challenge for this healing journey, and nothing less will do. To see your light. To embrace your light. To be brave and step over your fear to accept what your family and community and world needs you to do: exude your light all around you.

---

[10] Think this is just an indulgent, touch-feely exercise? Think again! This practice is based on the very real science of neuroplasticity, a part of our human experience we can tap into and make important use of. We'll explore this in more detail in chapter eight: DISCOVER.

As Marianne Williamson famously wrote in *A Return to Love*, "Your playing small does not serve the world."[11] Sound harsh? It's a clear call to action and recognition that how we understand ourselves and live our lives affects everyone: *you* need to love yourself, and *we* all need that too. Your light is necessary for your healing, and we're counting on your light, joined with our own, to heal our world.

Self-Love Action Steps

Remember, self-love is a verb—it's what you do that will engender the change you're looking for. Lay down your stories of unworthiness, of being less important than the rest, or not having enough time to squeeze yourself in. Get to work. Start with these simple practices right now.

Show Up for Yourself

Remember your list of three things you already do for yourself? Whatever those actions are, expand them. Allow yourself fifteen extra minutes of sleep in the morning. Take a short walk over your lunch break. Call someone you love. Write something. Plan a healthy meal. Hug your dog. It doesn't matter what you do. Start somewhere. Start small. Start with three. Write them down and start right now.

Make Yourself a Top Priority

You are as important as everything and everyone else in your life. You belong on your schedule just as much as they do. Don't let a single day pass without placing yourself front and center on your calendar. Be as militant about keeping those commitments to yourself as you are about keeping commitments to others. Everything else can wait. Make sure

---

[11] Marianne Williamson. *A Return to Love*. 1996.

HEAL KARYN SHANKS MD

that whatever you plan to do for yourself does not always get scheduled at the end of your day. Try putting yourself first. Go on, open your calendar and schedule yourself in.

Celebrate Yourself

That's right: celebrate, brag, pat yourself on the back. For doing this work. For all of your achievements. Just because you are awesome. What do you think happens when your mind and heart soak in that appreciation? You got it—they expand, they rise, they soar! Think of something you totally rock at and write it down or say it out loud!

Break the Rules

Be disobedient! There's no more profound way to honor yourself and who you are. You get to decide what's right for you. The way everyone else does things may not be for you. What they think of you for being who you are is not your concern (and you are none of their business!). Honor your needs and factor them into your decisions. Stop trying to please others all the time!

Practice Balance

Life isn't meant to be all work. Let yourself incorporate rest into your day. Create needed balance on your own terms. That may take the form of an electronics-free time in your day, limiting the number of times you check email, or turning off all notifications on your phone. It may be a short nap or a walk. Try driving, eating, or shopping without simultaneously talking on your cell phone. Turn your phone off entirely. Find ways to honor your need to be at peace, to focus on just one thing at a time, and to pause by pulling back and letting go.

Insist on Love

Surround yourself with people who affirm your worth and who are kind to you. Minimize your time with people who devalue you or make you feel uncomfortable. You may have toxic coworkers, bosses or friends. You can't completely avoid some of these people, but protect yourself by affirming your worth and minimizing contact with them. Change what you can. Know that you deserve to be fully loved and supported by the people around you. A friend of mine used to work with some tough people. She took to carrying or wearing a talisman and would touch it periodically throughout the day to remind herself of her strength.

Tell a New Story of Self-Love

Strengthen your mind pathways for self-love by working with affirmations that support it. Affirm gratitude for yourself. Do this whether you *feel* it or not. The practice will ultimately shift how you feel.

> *I am enough.*
> *I love myself.*
> *I am worthy.*
> *I believe in myself.*
> *I am a blessing to this world.*

If you find negative self-talk competing for space in your mind, substitute one of these affirmations. Write them on sticky notes and keep them where you can frequently see them to remind you. As you look at them, take pause. Let the words wash over you. Feel them. Then, live your self-love. Live like you love yourself.

WE LOVE OTHERS

And yes, of course, we love others. Once we've prioritized self-love, we can extend our focus to loving others. Love of one another is also an essential nutrient of our lives. Our families, children, lovers, and friends. Our communities. Our favorite authors, social icons, and heroes. We love them. And it is essential to our highest wellbeing to participate fully in this love.

Just like self-love, love to others is fundamentally in what we do. The big things. The small things. The whispers. The touch. Love is the kinetic energy of our actions, not the gooey puffed-up platitudes of Hollywood or Madison Avenue. It's real stuff. And it heals. Our love of others heals them. It heals our world. It all circles back to heal us.

The Heart's Call to Duty

Part of our social wiring is to be of service to others. Volunteerism has been shown to lead us to longer lives, while enjoying increased functional ability, decreased pain, and greater wellbeing. It promotes a sense of purpose and feelings of social connection for us as well as those we serve. Many studies have shown that people who volunteer their time to help others are happier and healthier compared to those who don't.

There are countless ways we can give of ourselves to benefit others. And it's often the simplest of acts that are the most transformative. One of the clerks at my grocery store always makes a point to remember my name and say, "Hi, Karyn! How are you?" It never fails to make my day. I make a special point to look for her and get in her checkout line. Her kindness and personal touch lifts all of us up.

The Leader Dogs for the Blind Prison Puppies Initiative

The Leader Dogs for the Blind, founded in 1939, is a one hundred percent philanthropically funded organization providing guide dogs and training to visually impaired clients free of charge to support lives of confidence, safety, and independence. The organization created an innovative Prison Puppies Initiative to address both the rising need for service dogs (for blind and disabled) and the void in meaningful rehabilitation for inmates incarcerated in medium to high security correctional facilities. While there was some apprehension about including prisoners—many of whom had been convicted of violent crimes, some serving life sentences—the program was launched in Iowa in 2002. The program leaders were hoping the initiative would provide dogs with ideal conditions for intensive training—twenty-four-hour care givers and trainers in peaceful, controlled settings—while providing the men with a sense of purpose through care for the animals.

The initiative has been a huge success, now expanded to eleven facilities throughout the Midwest, and it won the Mutual of America foundation's 2013 Community Partnership award.

The dogs are trained for a full year before becoming the eyes for and constant companions of their human partners. The puppies are brought into the prison and placed in the care of a single inmate who is responsible for their care and training 24-7, while being monitored and mentored by the staff of the prison and the Leader Dogs program.

The success of the program has been astounding. The puppies raised by inmates have a higher chance of graduating the program with its rigorous standards than those raised elsewhere in the community. This is thought to be due to the intensive nature of the work between inmates and dogs, the additional time the inmates have to spend with them, and the special passion the inmates have for the responsibility, companionship, and opportunity to serve others in a meaningful way.

The inmates benefit by closely bonding with the dogs and experiencing a sense of profound purpose in doing something important for someone else. They take great pride in their accomplishments, even competing with one another for the most well-behaved dogs. Inmates have expressed finding "inner peace," "doing something good finally," experiencing a "rare opportunity to help someone else," and helping others enjoy life as "an awesome thing."

This program has demonstrated how some of the most hardened and isolated members of our society find purpose and flourish when given the chance to give to others in a meaningful way.

Love of Others Supports Our Innate Need for Purpose

The inmate's responses in the Leader Dogs initiative demonstrate how we are wired for purpose. And purpose is inextricably connected to love: to belonging, connection, and service to others. Purpose doesn't have to be grandiose. It doesn't have to lift us off our feet. It can stem from the simple things in life that fill us up and connect us.

Viktor Frankl, who wrote *Man's Search for Meaning* after surviving Nazi concentration camps in the Second World War, observed that his fellow prisoners became sick and died after losing their sense of purpose, whether that meant living for their loved ones or contributing to the simple matters of community and self-care possible even within such harrowing conditions. He recognized that people lived longer when they had a greater will to live and actively sought out ways to cultivate connection and purpose in their everyday lives.

The many studies looking at the health benefits of living with purpose have shown reduced levels of stress and longer lives. It doesn't matter what lends that sense of purpose, though it's always about connection. It can be a deep sense of calling, a connection to a higher power, or simply tending purposefully to daily chores.

CREATE SPACE FOR LOVE

So how do we build on all this and actually generate concrete change in our lives? As Rumi reminded us, the love is there; we just need to remove the barriers. I say we need to create space for love. But love isn't easy for some of us, and it can take practice. With that in mind, we practice forgiveness. We practice gratitude. We practice receiving love.

Forgive

> *"You cannot forgive just once, forgiveness is a daily practice."*

> —*Sonia Rumzi*

In order to create space for love, we need to talk about the biggest creator of space there is: forgiveness. So, let me tell you a story about forgiveness.

My Forgiveness Story

It took me a long time to forgive my dad—to *truly* forgive him. The details of our relationship are not so important. What is important is that nothing he did or didn't do was actually about me, not ever. Over the years, I created many stories to explain to myself why he behaved as he did. Those stories always painted me as the victim. As I grew and matured in my thinking, I realized that I really like who I am and feel deeply blessed in my life. That doesn't mean I haven't struggled or suffered. But it does mean, ultimately, that my past—and my dad—played a very important part in my success as a human being.

And my stories were just that—stories. They were built upon my assumptions about what he thought, intended, believed—all things I couldn't possibly have known for certain. While he may have had deficiencies in his ability to connect in a loving way with his daughter, that's all I really know. With only behavior to go by, I created stories to fill in the blanks. Those stories may have protected me by helping me survive back then. But as I grew and matured, they no longer supported me.

This shift in my perspective about how to think about my relationship with my dad, as well as with others with whom I've struggled, has been singularly freeing: I get to choose my own life story. My daughter-father story could be all about abandonment and mean spiritedness, but its much more life affirming to make it a story about one person's ignorance and anxiety and the other rising up.

After fifteen years of no contact, my dad's wife invited me to visit him because his health was declining. He was developing dementia, and they had moved into a more supportive environment. To my surprise, I felt ready to go. I went with an open heart and mind. No expectations. No grudges. I worked deeply with the concept of my past with him not being personal.

As I sat with them during my visit, he didn't inquire about me, or the important things in my life, like my children, but it didn't feel personal. It didn't hurt me. It was completely about him. Yet we connected in a strange, though meaningful and purposeful way. I felt nothing but compassion for him as a human being struggling with great loss. He had changed so much. We'll never be close like a father and daughter perhaps should. There simply is no legacy of shared loving experience for that. I'll never get to experience the unconditional love of an adoring father. But he's my dad. He needs me now. All is forgiven.

Forgiveness Opens the Door to Love

Forgiveness is one of the biggest doorways to love. Forgiveness is when we release our stories about the past—stories that can stand in the way of love—and our *attachment* to them. It frees us and opens us to new connections and experiences.

Bad things happen. Elements of these events can be so profound and hurtful that the wounds come upon us without our bidding and without our stopping to decipher what happened. Like tripping on a rock and hitting our head. It happened. It hurt and there were ramifications. But we can release our attachment to the event. And we must. Forgiveness is our way of releasing the past and letting go of the need to have had events unfold in a different way.

We forgive for ourselves. It's not for the person we are forgiving. It's not pretending that our past didn't exist. We just don't let it define who we are. And yet, strangely and magically, when we gift ourselves with forgiveness and release the past, we do open up the possibility of healing for all concerned.

In the end forgiveness softens us. It opens the way for us to love ourselves more deeply as we realize that we were never the true target of our past. Forgiveness opens our hearts, frees us, and makes us ripe for the infinite possibilities of our lives that would not have been possible otherwise. The energy we used for remembering, fuming, and hurting becomes available for something new—our growth and recovery. Numerous studies have shown that forgiveness is good for our health: it lowers our stress response, inflammation, risk for heart disease, blood pressure, and levels of depression and anxiety. Forgiveness is vital medicine.

Be Grateful

A grateful life takes a lot of work, even when there is so much to be grateful for. Our stresses and traumas can tether our focus to what upsets us, needs to be fixed, or has to be done. It's how our brains were designed—to keep us alive and in working order. It's so easy to forget what makes us blessed and lucky, though if we look closely, our lives are filled to the brim with fortunate things.

Practicing gratitude does not mean that we have to pretend to be thankful for what is bad for us. It doesn't mean that the challenges disappear. We don't dismiss the importance of the toxic elements of our lives that also need to be excised. We simply remember and amplify what is good.

For many of us, experiencing adversity helps crystallize appreciation for the positive aspects of our lives. We are reminded of how precious life is. A challenging past can lead to a happier present. Studies show that people currently experiencing adversity may not be able to access gratitude in the present, but after working through the negative events, are more appreciative of what's good and have a deepened sense of life's preciousness.

Gratitude practice expands our mind space for what's good, creating much needed balance for our "worst-case scenario" brains. And it's not just a hippie's fantasy. It's real stuff—science-y stuff: neural networks, mind pathways, epigenetics. Our thoughts create our reality.

Gratitude has enormous health benefits. Studies link it to greater optimism, reduced stress, less depression, better general health, and increased longevity. Patients with heart failure who kept a gratitude journal experienced better sleep, reduced inflammation, less depressed mood and fatigue, and better self-efficacy to maintain cardiac function. Gratitude practice bolsters our immunity, lowers blood pressure, and leads to greater happiness and spiritual connection. Gratitude drives generosity and compassion for others and reduces loneliness.

Receive Love: Risk Being Your True Self

> "The practice of love offers no place of safety. We risk loss, hurt, pain. We risk being acted upon by forces outside our control."
>
> —bell hooks, All About Love: New Visions

Love is so pure in its expression and intention that it is a window into our whole, true, authentic selves. This can be terrifying. Brené Brown, author of *Daring Greatly*, teaches that exposing our true selves to others reveals where we are most vulnerable, but is the only path to "openheartedness." Armoring our hearts to protect ourselves from pain removes our accessibility to love and connection. But showing others difficult emotions, like guilt, shame, and fear, connects us more deeply and invites their more authentic selves to meet ours.

This is hard stuff. What makes us feel vulnerable is what brings us to our knees. But vulnerability, according to Brown's research, is the only path to courage and openheartedness. *The only path to receiving love.* We have to expose who we really are, *be* our true selves, scars and all, to become available for love.

Step over your fear and practice being who you truly are. Dare to let others see you. Put your toe in the water. Work toward full immersion.

FOUR LOVE PRACTICES

Practice Letting Love In

The givers and nurturers—you know who you are. So good at giving you forget to get a little for yourself. Not a sustainable way to live and thrive, is it? Your tank needs to be filled too. This may be strenuous work for some, and scary (it has been for me), yet profound. Here are some of the gifts we can give to ourselves (as well as others!) when we let the love in:

- Accept that compliment. Say "thank you," and don't deflect. Just accept it.

- Let those who offer help you—practice saying, "yes."

- Ask for help! Take a deep breath and jump off that cliff. You'll survive. And guess what? They'll either say "yes," or "no." If you keep at it you'll find there are many helpful hands out there, and they'll feel honored that you asked.

- Don't put off creating that healing team any longer—schedule appointments with everyone you need—the massage therapist, chiropractor, acupuncturist, nutritionist, counselor, and so on. You deserve their help in your self-care.

Practice Amplifying Love

> *"You don't need to justify your love, you don't need to explain your love, you just need to practice your love. Practice creates the master."*
>
> —*Miguel Ruiz, The Mastery of Love: A Practical Guide to the Art of Relationship*

Love is exquisitely physical. The emotions and sensations of love are tangible as they live and are felt within the body. We can feel love's energy and hear its wisdom. Even the HeartMath researchers were able to measure its physical effects and benefits.

Knowing love is physical makes it more accessible to us. We can feel it, hear it, speak it, create it, and move it around. You experienced love's physical sensations as you thought about someone or something you loved in our earlier exercise. That simple practice allowed you ready access to the positive benefits of love. What else can we do to amplify love?

- Acts of kindness.

- Affirm love.

- Love meditation (The following exercise is one of my favorite practices for expanding love in the body.)

- Hug.

- Kiss.

- Have sex (good sex, with someone you feel safe with).

Exercise: Breathe in Love, Breathe out Negativity

This is an exercise for which you'll need a few minutes of quiet and a comfortable seat. Come back to it later if you must. But do come back—it's worth it!

Sit seated with your eyes closed, hands over heart. Breathe deeply and let it all go. Think about who or what you love most, like we did in our earlier exercise. Allow that sensation of love to arrive and expand within you. Continue to breathe slowly and deeply and concentrate on that person or thing you love and the physical sensations it creates.

Are there negative emotions or sensations competing for your attention? There might be anger, hurt, grief, anxiety, frustration, depression, pain, discomfort—emotions or sensations that also reside within the body, that get in the way of your perception and experience of love.

As you sit quietly, breathe in love. Imagine that your breath is the golden light of love coming in through the crown of your head as you inhale. Feel or see it descend, flowing in with your breath, filling up your chest. Then let that golden light of love expand within you on the exhale.

Imagine the competing negative emotions or sensations (pain, frustration, grief, anxiety, anger?) as black smoke. Let your next inhale push that black smoke down through your body, letting it leave through the base of your spine and enter the earth.

Breathe in the golden light of love through the crown of your head. Breathe out, let it expand. Breathe in, push that black smoke of negativity down and out through the base of the spine. Breathe out, see it leave and enter the earth.

I like to think that the earth "composts" that pain or negative energy, reutilizing it for something good.

Say: "Golden light of love in" as you inhale and exhale. Then, "dark smoke of [fill in the blank; for example, negativity] out" on the next inhale and exhale. Repeat ten times.

How do you feel? Is there a detectible shift?

I have used this simple breath visualization technique on difficult emotions that were too painful for me to take on with my mind. It's easy to get tangled up in our stories about the nature of hurt feelings, grief, or anxiety. With this simple technique, we can bypass trying to mentally work things out and release a lot of the negative energy being held within the body.

There are times for all of us when the simplest way to work on love and the negative emotions that get in its way, is to go directly to the body, where we can work with the emotional energy of love, bypassing our stories that get in the way. (We'll discuss mind and stories more in chapter eight.)

Practice Being Grateful

There are always things to be grateful for even on the darkest, dreariest, most depressing, lonely, or stressful days. Remember that you need not *feel* grateful to practice and reap the benefits.

- Make a list of ten things you are grateful for, whether you feel grateful or not. There is always something to express gratitude about: My bed is soft and warm. The beauty of that tree. My car is in good working order. The warmth of the sun against my skin. I have indoor plumbing. Do this now and repeat daily.

- Think of someone you love—a child, partner, parent, or pet. Let your thoughts of them fill your heart. Think of them and breathe into your heart, expressing gratitude for them.

- Think of someone or a situation that challenges you. Consider the benefits of being challenged—how it expands you, teaches you, makes you stronger and more resilient. Express your gratitude for that person or situation whether you feel it or not. Then see how that challenge shifts in a more positive direction.

- Is there someone in your life who you feel grateful for right now? Tell them. Even if you're feeling too scared to do it now, say it out loud or write it: I am grateful for you.

- Learn to receive expressions of gratitude from others. Next time someone thanks you, rather than deflecting it away ("Oh, that was nothing!"), accept it fully.

Practice Softening the Harsh Edges

When we soften our hard, rough, defensive edges, we open ourselves to love and the more tender aspects of life.

While a juicy meltdown may feel satisfying when life gets too overwhelming, we always regret it, don't we? It never leads to a positive, constructive resolution. There's inevitably fallout that leaves us feeling crappy. It takes us far away from love.

My instant go-to is a powerful trick learned from my yoga teacher many years ago. I call it the art of softening.

Soften. Soften your body, soften your face, soften your skin, soften your mind, soften your expectations, soften your stories. I hear her voice, even today, as I confront a challenge. I hear it when I'm worrying, becoming frustrated about something, having trouble falling to sleep, or judging myself. It works in an instant, separating me from worry or tyrannical stories. It requires no thought. And it makes everything, well . . . softer.

Try it. When you hear your own critical voice—the one that knows so completely, exactly how you've screwed up, or how impossible it all is, how unfair things are—ignore it and instead say, "Soften." And breathe.

One simple word. Note how the edges of those limiting thoughts begin to blur, how they become less sharp. How the certainty, judgment, and hopelessness begin to fade. Feel the possibilities of what could be flow into that space you've created for them. The room you've made for inspiration, wisdom, creativity, resolution, and of course, love.

Softening doesn't mean total surrender, giving up, or walking away from your troubles. It's just a compassionate way to walk into your troubles, open to a fresh perspective.

LAST THOUGHTS

Now that you've created space for healing by letting go and have stepped up to love (especially for yourself!), it's time to find, trust, and live from your strong, resilient center. Join me on the next part of our journey—the adventure of creating balance.

Chapter Four

BALANCE

Find Your Strong Center and Become Stress Resilient

We've created space. We've welcomed love. Now we find, nurture, and strengthen our center—our sacred home, the place of rest and strength within us that both soothes and energizes.

From this core—our anchor—we explore the challenges, struggles, and joys of our lives. We let them shape us, and energize us, as we rise and let go, rise and let go. Like breath, like the beating of our hearts, this pulse of our lives is the rhythm of our genius and the balance that energizes our healing.

TO STAY ON YOUR FEET—TO THRIVE—YOU MUST FIND YOUR STRONG CENTER

Our center is us. It's who we are at our very core—our inner wiser self, our soul. From this center we navigate and negotiate our lives. It guides and gives us strength to fully engage with all that life brings us—the challenges, the joys, and the daily chores. And in its wisdom, it draws us back for rest, reflection, and renewal. We must nourish this center of ours to remain strong, wise, and resilient.

How about when we're sick or depleted of energy? In our weakened state it's easy to lose touch with our center. It's hard to reach out to face life's challenges when we're physically or emotionally struggling. But your center is there, filled to the brim with untapped potential. And you can find it. You can support it and make it strong again.

Balance and Me

I only understand balance—*really* understand it—when I bump up against the harsh edges of *im*balance. The overwhelm and weariness that make it clear I've taken on too much. The loss of energy, time, or focus to take it *all on right now*. This is the price I pay for being a curious, passionate, and excitable person. I want to know it all. Do it all. Try it all. Right now.

The wisdom of my center reminds me of my limits, calling me back to rest, restore, and rethink my life strategy. What do I need to let go of? How must I change my focus? How do I need to strengthen and renew?

Here's what I've learned: what's most important when I feel out of balance is that I come back to my center and take a careful listen. I let go of the frustration I inevitably feel about falling out of balance. It's just unavoidable. Sometimes it feels bad, and I'm overwhelmed. Sometimes it feels good, and I'm exploring new things. But any extreme for too long is depleting.

But balance is not about being relaxed and calm and placid all the time. It's about continuing to live to the fullest while listening and heeding the lessons and creating a resilient center from which to engage life with strength. Like my yoga teacher says, "Hug in first, then extend out." Or my trainer who reminds me, "Engage your core first, then lift that heavy weight." Step out—heck, *leap* out there—but do so from a strong resilient center, always prepared to hug back in.

And always remember that balance is not the fantasyland of everything-just-so. It's way messier (and more wonderful) than that. What we're going to work on here is a strong core that you can trust to heal you and pull you back when you're hurting, but that also lets you fully explore the wonders that life has in store for you.

Balance is How We Engage with Our Lives

Balance is not a static point in the trajectory of our lives at which we triumphantly arrive when we've finally gotten it all together. No, it's a dynamic force within us. It's a rhythmic push-pull, leaning in and stepping back, rising up and taking pause. This rhythm reflects how our center is always evaluating, adjusting, and responding to who we are, what challenges us, and what we need at every moment.

In science we call this dynamic balance *homeostasis*, or *equilibrium*. It's not an option—it's simply how the natural world works. Every biological system achieves a certain balance between the needs, stresses, and resources of its circumstances. Increased rainfall makes the river run faster and wider, and the plants grow new leaves and bloom. Decrease the rainfall, and the plants curl their leaves to preserve water.

As humans, we're part of this very same world. Our bodies-minds-spirits will establish a balance based on our circumstances.

However, we have one key advantage over the rivers and plants—we have conscious choice. Rather than accepting a point of balance based on our current circumstances, we can work to change the circumstances that influence it. We have the opportunity to intentionally nourish and strengthen our center to create a dynamic vitality. We get to actively, *purposefully* engage with our lives in ways that are more durable and that direct our equilibrium to support how we choose to live.

What is Healthy Balance?

So, what does healthy balance feel like in our real everyday lives? Of course, that answer will vary from one person to the next. Risk takers and thrill seekers might feel dissatisfied with what the quiet homebody feels quite content with. But we can still generalize some ideas about what balanced lives have:

- enough energy to live lives that make us happy,

- enough internal fire to follow our curiosity or go after our dreams,

- strength and resilience in the midst of life's changes and challenges,

- ability to manage stress well, without depleting ourselves,

- ability to manage time well, without the sense of rushing all the time,

- a strong sense of self—who we are, what we believe, what we want,

- ability to maintain strong personal protective boundaries.

Self-Reflective Exercise: What Healthy Balance Feels Like

How does healthy balance feel in your life?

First, write down three areas of your life that you balance well. These should be parts of your life that you feel good about how you are managing.

Then, list three areas of your life in which you feel out of balance.

Compare and contrast your two lists. What can you learn from one that you can apply to the other?

For example, I have great balance in many self-care arenas of my life, particularly when it comes to food, sleep, meditation, and movement. I have a structure I follow—a food plan that fits my needs, a sleep routine, a daily meditation practice, and scheduled opportunities for movement and exercise. I need these things, and I've found the right formula that takes care of me. But in my creative life as a writer, I get over focused, obsessive, and can have too many projects going at once, leading to overwhelm. The overwhelm is teaching me to moderate this part of my life, as I already have with the domains that I do well with. And like those other domains, I've learned I need a structure to follow—like working on just one project at a time, allowing rest periods, and accepting delays as a necessary part of my creative process. It's all a work in progress.

CENTER GEOGRAPHY: OUR INTERNAL POINT OF BALANCE

Like the center point of a compass rose, *our* center is the internal point of balance—physical, emotional, and spiritual—from which we engage with every aspect of our lives.

It occupies tangible physical space within our bodies and also resides in our inner emotional-energetic intelligent consciousness. Like all aspects of ourselves, these dimensions of our core center are intimately intertwined. What we do to strengthen any one dimension of our center strengthens the whole. When we talk about the body—as we will extensively in this chapter—we're really talking about the whole package. When we go into the body, we're also going into the soul.

Physically, our core center is the hub for the physical strength and physiological processes that support our energy. It helps us blast out fuel when we need to do something big. It regulates the essential life-sustaining functions that go on automatically (energy production, circulation, breath, sleep). It is the structural and functional center of our bodies—the muscles, connective tissue, and internal vigor of our core that supports our position in space and movement through the physical realm of our lives.

Mentally and spiritually, we experience our core as our "inner self"—the space of our inner strength and wisdom, our small quiet voice. Our soul. It's our anchor, our sacred home, the wise inner fire we can trust to guide and support us.

If our center is the core from which we establish equilibrium, how do we create balance? Well, we start by building a strong center.

BUILD YOUR STRONG CENTER

We build a strong center to create balance—the dynamic equilibrium that supports us in everything. To do this we must:

- Find and connect to it.

- Protect it.

- Nourish it.

- Challenge it.

Find and Connect to Your Strong Center

Listen quietly, and you'll sense your center.

Many of us have lost touch with our center. It often becomes lost as we shift our attention and allegiance to the "experts" in our families and culture, feeling they know more than we do. Or we're seduced by the false cultural promises of "easy," "fast," "simple," or "certain." We may have forgotten that we're the captains of our ships. Or we've suffered, and in our suffering, we've lost our awareness of it.

But whether you're aware of it or not, your center is there.

Let's find it. Daily practice will solidify your knowledge about having a center, and help you begin a relationship with it that is tangible, accessible, and reliable. As you experience its location within you and learn to trust its strength and wisdom, your center becomes ... *you.* Your core. Who you are. No longer just a place of refuge, you'll learn to inhabit it and live your life from it.

Exercise: Find Your Center with Breath

Let's take an expedition to that center of yours. Let's find it so you'll know where to go when you need to tap into its strength. First, let's stand well: bare feet on the ground, your feet approximately hip-distance apart. Squeeze your buttocks just a bit and tilt your pelvis forward while engaging your abdominal muscles. Open your chest, stick your heart out, and flip your hands so palms face forward. Let your arms dangle at your sides, shoulders back, allow your shoulder blades to slide down your back.

Breathe slowly and deeply in and out. Feel your breath expand within you with each inhale. Allow an audible sigh on the exhale. Stand tall. Now, place your hands over your midsection, just on or above your belly button and under your ribs. Become aware of your core. Breathe in deeply here. This is your center. Pause and memorize this image, this feeling, this emotion of this place inside you. This is your core. Your center. The place of strength and wisdom within you. This is you. See and feel it. Feel the comfort of it as you breathe deeply into it.

Pause here for as long as you like and continue to breathe deeply in and out of your core center. And listen: Do you hear anything? Any whispers? Words? Messages? If you don't hear anything this time, don't worry. Introduce yourself to your center and be sure to come back soon!

Practices for Strengthening Your Strong Center

Once you've found your center, there are simple ways you can stay in touch with it and continue to strengthen it through daily practice. Connecting to your strong center calls you to be still, feel, and listen.

Breathe. Allow your breath to navigate you straight to your center. Conscious breathing slows you down, diminishes distractions, and helps you feel and hear your center and its still quiet voice. Repeat the simple breath exercise we just did. Take a few deep, mindful breaths into your center throughout your day.

Meditate. Meditation does not have to be a prescribed esoteric practice, it does not require a guru (you are your own guru—it's your wise center), and it can be most anything that you simply do mindfully, quietly, and without distraction. Done reverently and with deep presence, doing the laundry and mowing the lawn are meditation practices.

Daily meditation is a beautiful and effective way to connect to your center and prepare you for engaging with what's to come in your day in a more balanced way.

You might choose a moving meditation—a quiet walk in the woods, a yoga practice, or a mindfully executed workout in the gym. A quiet seated meditation is also suitable and allows for the deeper quiet and focus that many of us desire in our meditation, using a variety of techniques: breath work, mantras, affirmations, prayers, and visualization.

Choose a meditation style that suits you. Commit to it every day. Begin with baby steps. Three to five minutes first thing in the morning using a smart phone meditation app is a beautiful way to start. Gradually increase your time as you go. Use briefer versions of your meditation to help relieve stress of a difficult day—one or two breaths during a bathroom break will help you greatly. Your center will be grateful for the check-in.

Laugh. Cultivate humor in the face of challenge. It allows us to instantly diffuse the negative impact of stress within our bodies and minds. Laughter shakes our cores (literally), releases tension, and mobilizes resources we need to engage with our challenging situations. I love how author Anne Lamott describes laughter as "carbonated holiness." Laughter is a sure indication that we don't take ourselves too seriously and allows us to punch through negative aspects of stress, getting us closer to the transformation we need to move through difficult times.

Self-Reflection Exercise: Humor

There was a lot of gallows humor that helped us release some of the stress of medical school and residency training. Likewise, our favorite comedians go after all people and situations for the sake of humor. They give us a healthy sense of proportion when we take things too seriously. Laughter helps us release the powerful energy of our life experiences. Can you find any funny elements, particularly about yourself, in any of your current challenges? You may need to stretch to find them, but I promise you they're there. Seen in the right light, we're all pretty hilarious. Let laughter lighten your load.

Protect Your Strong Center

Once we've connected with and strengthened our center, we must also be prepared to protect it. It's so easy to take some things for granted, especially ourselves—a key theme we've explored before. There are so many things in our lives we work hard to protect that we can forget to protect ourselves!

How do we protect our center? Many of these are common themes we've talked about: self-love, simplifying and relieving distraction, and healing guilt and shame. We've also got to protect our center from powerlessness and burnout. Addressing these potent strength-sappers creates more room for risk taking and pursuing our passions.

Protect Your Center from Feeling Powerless: Trust Yourself

Being confronted with life challenges without a sense of control over the outcome leads to persistently high stress. Case in point: my internship and residency in internal medicine were nightmarish at times, with nights on call, thirty-six-hour work shifts, and life and death situations to manage—sometimes alone. But what helped me was to frame it in the understanding that I made the conscious choice to be there. There was a larger goal and purpose for me in spite of the difficult conditions, and there were important ways in which I was supported through the process. It was still traumatizing at times, but I kept my sights on the higher purpose.

My own equilibrium swung from days of wondering why I was putting myself through this to days of amazing connections with grateful patients whom I was able to help and learn from. But through it all, my center was strong. It was my anchor. It gave me peace and direction every day. I had to move through that world, but it was my center that guided me.

Self-Reflection Exercise: Use the Strength of Your Core

Let's pause to take another quick expedition into your strong center. Think of one of your own challenging situations. Then think about the strong center of your body. How can you use that core to empower you in the midst of that situation? You don't have to take control of the situation or walk away from it (unless that's how your inner wisdom guides you). But can you find some aspect of your situation—a higher purpose, a goal, a hoped-for outcome that resonates with your core? That sustains and strengthens you?

Protect Your Center from Burnout, While Making Room for Passion and Grit

Burnout can occur when we've not adequately supported our core. Passion, creativity, and genius all require energy and resources to sustain them. For instance, I get excited about a project I am working on, and then think about it all the time, use every available nook and cranny in my life to work on it. I am usually driven by passion and excitement. But I can suddenly feel tired, weak, and wimpy—burned-out. This is when I know I've gone too far, that I've fueled my passion without replenishing my reserve of resources. But by listening to my center, I now read these signs from my body sooner. I recognize the imbalance before it goes too far. Sometimes the solution is rest, other times it's to find a new strategy.

It helps to know our great accomplishments don't have to be done alone. I recently heard an epic talk on the origin of burnout by Dr. Joan Borysenko, a widely acclaimed mind-body psychologist and researcher, in which she explored the roots of burnout and found it is often driven by a passionate sense of service to others. She recommended that we tap into "soul Universal energy" rather than our bodies' more limited supply of "adrenal energy." In other words, we need to know it's not all up to us. We can trust the universe or our trusted champions for support and take care to replenish the resources we utilize in our efforts. (We'll get back to the adrenals in a bit.)

Nourish Your Strong Center

You've now become acquainted with your strong center. You know how to connect to it and protect it. But like all living things, it also needs to be nurtured and nourished to make it strong and resilient.

Nourish Your Center by Creating Resilience through Self-Care

That is what you've shown up here for. It's everything you're learning and practicing from this book. Self-care works by building resilience—the strength and resources we need to successfully face the many challenges of our lives.

Nourish Your Center by Literally Strengthening Your Core

One of the easiest, quickest, and most accessible ways to strengthen your center is to engage your physical core. This can be done by moving more in a vertical position (as simple as sitting less). That's right—*strengthen* your core. Engage it, squeeze it, lift it, hold it, and let it stabilize you.

Work with a pro: learn yoga or Pilates, or work with a good trainer at the gym. They all will train you to find, focus, and strengthen your core safely. Then use it throughout your life—move more, stand and sit well, walk with strength, hug more tightly.[12] Stand tall, strong, and wise from your beautiful strong center.

Nourish Your Center by Creating Strong Personal Boundaries

Actively standing your ground and saying "no," when necessary, amplifies the energy of your center.

- Say, "no" when you mean no.

- Check your assumptions about what will happen as a result of saying "no."

- Be willing to stand alone (but tall and proud) if you feel like the only one saying "no."

- Give up playing "nice." Nice isn't the truth, right? Nice can kill you.13

---

[12] More on healthy movement practices in chapter six, MOVE.

[13] We'll explore "nice" as a strategy to manage difficult emotions in chapter nine, FLOW.

Nourish Your Center by Creating Equanimity

My client Linda has suffered crushing blows to her health, her vitality, and her sense of self over many years of illness from persistent Lyme disease and coinfections. She has spent months barely able to get out of bed due to fatigue and pain. But she is the fiercest warrior in the face of illness I have ever witnessed.

What does she do? Quite simply, she never gives up. She keeps the faith. She mobilizes her team of experts and supporters. If solutions aren't apparent, she moves on to discover someone else who can help her. She asks her friends, neighbors, and fellow church members for help, which they gladly do. Perhaps most importantly, she wakes up every single day with a dogged determination to live her best life—even if that means spending the day in bed—and to find the meaning even on the darkest days. She would be the first one to say that in spite of her suffering her life is rich beyond measure. I bow to her.

Resilient people, like Linda, are able to thrive in the face of stress, challenge, catastrophe, or whatever life throws at them. They fall down. They experience devastation. But they don't give up or let what happens to them define who they are. They are able to embrace the uncertainties of life and see setbacks or crises as opportunities. They are challenged by failure but remain undaunted—they don't give up. They embrace change and know that it's okay to release control.

Who are these flexible people who can maintain a balanced life even through the trials of stressful times and extraordinary situations while many of us struggle? What do they have?

Resilient people are the most successful at living and being happy because they have built a reserve of *equanimity*—the ability to stay calm in the face of stress and to engage with life's challenges without becoming overwhelmed by them. They have a reservoir of personal skills, attributes, and practices that help them stay balanced when faced with a challenge. Equanimity is their antidote to the barrage of stressors that come at them constantly. Stress is just as much a part of their lives as it is for all of us, but their attitudes and practices in the face of stress support them and help them maintain a strong center.

Equanimity can be learned. It comes about from the practice of present-moment awareness that we explore throughout this book: awareness of ourselves, our bodies and their sensations, and what's around us right now, in this moment. This simple presence—a focus on what's in this moment right now, not the past or future, not our stories or other distractions—allows us to be fully available to the good things that are happening right now, in addition to the challenges and suffering. Presence allows us to access our strong center, keeping us in balance, and shifting us into a more positive perspective.

We can practice equanimity through presence by using all the exercises and practices we've discussed so far—mindful breathing, meditation, laughter— even while doing laundry, mowing the lawn, or cleaning the house. They all engage our awareness about what's real, right here, right now.

Equanimity Is Not Disengagement.

It is important to know that equanimity does not mean that we're all relaxed, all the time. It does not mean that we are disengaged. It's about flow, a balance of calm readiness with engagement and resourcefulness. Stress avoidance and excessive relaxation have a cost: missed opportunities, disengagement, isolation, and anxiety.

Take, for example, a client of mine, whom I will call Ben. Ben meditates for four hours every day. He is a natural introvert, suffers from anxiety, and finds great solace in this practice. He often goes on retreats and spends days to weeks in a meditative state. These practices ease his anxiety, but even so, he has trouble in his work, struggles to stay awake, and has a hard time engaging with coworkers and clients. He has no friends. He has vague ideas about creative projects but no initiative or motivation to even start on them.

Ben is not engaged in his life, and he is hardly aware of his body. He works hard in his meditation practice to transcend his painful emotions. His stated goal is "elevation," but in reality, his intensive meditation practice is his way of numbing himself and denying the wisdom of his emotions. While it is true that a number of the great meditation masters spend many hours in meditative or contemplative states, their goal is wisdom through embodiment, not escape from painful lives. What Ben actually accomplishes by leaving his body is temporary anesthesia, which ultimately exacerbates his anxiety and disconnects him from opportunities to receive guidance from his emotions.[14] His practice

---

[14] More about strategies we use to disconnect from challenging emotions in chapter nine, FLOW.

disconnects him from the people in his life who could provide him with comfort and support.

Equanimity Exercise: Open to Strength

Let's take a moment to practice equanimity in the face of challenge by tapping into the strength of your core. Think about a challenging or stressful experience in your life. Sink into it. Remember what it felt like. Can you feel your body responding to the mere memory of that stressful time or experience? Spend just thirty or so seconds immersing yourself in that memory to prepare you for a quick antidote.

Now, let's create a posture that engages the strength of your core: stand up, place your feet hip-distance apart, and feel your feet against the earth. Once again, squeeze your buttocks just a bit, tuck your pelvis for stability, and let your arms fall to your sides. Feel your chest open as you flip your palms to face forward. Standing here in this pose, take three deep cleansing breaths. Breathe in slowly, filling your entire torso and chest with air, then breath out, letting it all go, perhaps sighing and making noise with that exhalation.

After your three breaths, turn your face to look skyward and raise your arms up into the air, creating a large V. Relax your shoulders, let your shoulder blades release down your back, relax your face, and hold this position. Engage your abdominal muscles to stabilize your core as you continue to hold this pose. Continue to breathe deeply as you look to the sky, arms wide overhead, core strong, heart open. Spend about a minute in this pose—open to receive, open to strength.

Then, observe: What did you feel as you held this pose? Was there a shift from the stressful memory to something else? Perhaps calm, strength, confidence, fortification? Amy Cuddy, a psychologist who writes and speaks about the value of power poses, focuses on poses like this one in her book, Presence: Bringing Your Boldest Self to Your Biggest

Challenges, and her famous TED Talk. After just a minute or two of holding a power pose, there is a profound physiological shift from stress and anxiety to stress resilience—with lower cortisol and higher testosterone levels. People who practice power poses report a stronger sense of strength within themselves within seconds, They enjoy increased confidence, greater calm, and deeper engagement with what is happening in the moment.

This is a simple pose that you can do anywhere to shift the discomfort of stress or anxiety instantly through use of a positive, open posture into greater equanimity and control.

Nourish Your Center by Trusting the Flow of Life

We know that balance from a strong center will give us the strength and resilience to support our energy and healing. We want to drive forward and work hard to get that. We want to take control of it. But there's another side to that dynamic balance: we also have to trust in the flow of life.

My yoga teacher explains this as the dynamic of "effort versus ease" on our mats. It's the sweet spot that exists between exercising our willful ambitions and trusting in the flow of life. My trainer teaches essentially the same thing with his reminders for me to "coax the gains," neither under- or overdoing it. My goals will come, but there is a flow of which I'm a part and which I must honor.

We want to work hard, do our best, and get better. But many of us try to force it. That's not always what's best—it's excessive, it depletes resources, and leads to injury. All without the payoff we seek.

The balance is in pushing for our goals and ideals while allowing for the larger flow of life around us. Respecting it. Honoring it. Trusting it.

Challenge Your Strong Center

Of course, balance demands both equanimity and challenge. Challenging your center means inviting stress to become your wise teacher.

Whoa! Wait a minute. Say what? Invite stress? But I thought all this core strength and balance stuff was going to reduce my stress!

Indeed, it will, grasshopper. But it's always the *challenges* of life that make us grow strong. Hear me out, please!

We *must* engage our center with challenge: *we must have stress*. Challenge trains every aspect of who we are to keep us alive and thriving. Stress, stripped of its emotional context, is how we power ourselves to engage that challenge. The dread and overwhelm that stress can cause are stories—they're how we *perceive* stress. The stress itself, is a messenger and, simply put, is the biology of our center—it powers our life energy.

Yes, I'm trying to tell you that stress is good. In fact, stress is the genius of being human. Stress is all about the challenge we need to grow and learn and engage successfully with our lives. Stress supports the energy we must have to get up every day, to survive, and to be present for our lives—to slog through the muck, pursue our passions, and rise to our potential.

For the rest of this chapter we'll take a deep dive into stress—the ultimate challenge, feedback about how we're doing, and foundational source of our life energy.

STRESS: THE POWER OF OUR CORE

"Life is either a daring adventure or nothing at all."

—Helen Keller, The Open Door

My Beautiful Stressful Life

I have lived a stressful life. It hasn't been easy, but the stress has always led me to deep introspection, to wrestle with the challenges I've faced, to reflect on the meaning of things, and always to grow and become stronger. In this way, in a funny and unexpected twist on things, my stressful life has made me happy, grateful, and full to the brim with the richness and meaning of life.

It's curious how some of the most stressful times of my life—those that I worked hard to remedy and thought I'd never want to repeat again—are some of the same times I look back on now with soul-satisfying reminiscence, revisiting the intensity as well as the stories that have made my life beautiful.

I measure the success of my life by what fills me with meaning and purpose. And while I've had my share of trauma, difficulty, and pain there has always been some jewel of discovery. Perhaps in the way someone stepped up for me, or how I've connected to someone else, or the crucial lessons I learned about myself. It is in this way that my stressful life has been one big beautiful adventure, one that I can't imagine not having been a part of. Even the greatest difficulty has shaped me into who I am today.

The happiest period of my life, hands down, was also the most stressful—at times over-the-top, mind-blowingly stressful—when my husband and I were raising our young children. I recall the exhaustion, sleep deprivation, constant demands on our attention, worry about being good enough parents, total lack of downtime for ourselves. It was often a chaotic time of juggling, multitasking, and being present long past the hour when there was energy to stay alert and awake. We made life especially difficult for ourselves by creating guidelines for our parenting that we stuck to because it seemed better for our children, though terribly inconvenient for us—like no electronics on school nights unless it was specifically for a school project, or limiting exposure to television on the weekends so they'd be protected from the manipulation of advertisers. Like daily hands-on reading together, writing, puzzle doing, arts and crafts, and play that was fun and engaging (and exhausting). Like creating space to hang together every day no matter what.

Despite the stress it was one of the happiest times of my life, because it was all for love. Along with the stress and exhaustion of that precious time, came our children's smiles, raucous laughter, jokes, singing, creating, soul churning talks, the "big bed book club" every night, being together, living together, growing together. We created a beautiful life together. And they became our greatest teachers. I got to experience the world anew through their eyes. My cynical view of the world was forever blown apart by those magnificent angelic creatures, their hearts wide open, eyes wide open, exuding joy and optimism just for being, seeing and experiencing the best in everything. Every step was a miracle. And I'd do it all again. Every sacrifice was worth it.

I learned big lessons about myself, lessons I could not have learned another way. That my heart is infinite. That my love for my boys is a tsunami of emotion and devotion, and I can step up when called. I can step up to the day-to-day endless challenges of being there.

I can sacrifice my own interests in favor of the ones I love. I can do all that. And the decision to love is made all the more pointed and focused and energized by my sacrifices. I *chose* my boys.

My life has helped me understand the central message I want to convey here: beyond all the details about stress and what it is and how it affects us, *stress is good, stress is wise, stress is what makes life worth living.* Rather than killing me, which I was taught would happen if I sustained high levels of stress over long periods of time, it has energized me, ennobled me, filled my life in ways I would never have imagined. Because all of my stress has been about me *engaging* in my life: stepping up, committing, exploring, experimenting, failing, loving, creating, and living life to its fullest. And all the negative aspects of stress—the agony and exhaustion—have forced me to scrutinize my life and make it better, to become someone better, to live the life I was meant to live.

The Biological Purpose of Stress

Beyond the feelings associated with stress, stress is so much more, driving the energy, action, and learning that helps us engage successfully with all aspects of our lives. The discomfort of stress is what we tend to focus on, but that's actually *distress*, not the stress itself—at least biologically speaking. Biological stress is what we feel when the things that are important to us are challenged, fortifying us through our biology, to take meaningful action.

The strength and magnitude of our stress biology is determined by the size and significance of the challenge. This involves two main factors:

- to what degree the challenge matters to us, and

- how important it is for keeping us alive.

Our Feelings of Stress are Part of Its Biology

The uncomfortable *feelings* of stress—the tension or unhappiness we feel when there's too much going on, when the demands on us are high, or when we're uncomfortable about what is happening to us—are not meant to torture us. *These feelings are part of the purposefulness of stress.*

The pain tells us to move our hand away from the fire. The fear tells us to move away from that scary person. The discomfort of stress motivates us to change, to grow, to learn, to take action, to move ourselves away from what's not working and toward more harmony and balance in our lives.

Stress, in this way, is inherently linked to the *meaning* of our lives. We feel stress the most when things matter. And our stress systems ramp up to a greater degree when the big things are on the line—our survival, what we love, what means the most to us—all those things that can challenge us the most.

Stress Builds Resilience

In this way stress builds resilience. The more stress we experience, the greater potential we have for resilience. Depending on how we think about it, we get better at stress with practice. We often consider resilience to be the resistant stance we take in the face of stress, of how to confront or to *survive* stress. But, in truth, stress itself make us stronger, more fortified, smarter, and more capable of handling the future challenges of our lives through its elaborate biology (neurochemistry, hormones, energy systems) and psychology (learning, memory, emotional wisdom).

This doesn't mean we don't suffer or get thrown off balance, but stress resilience is how we get back up after falling and recover balance after a challenge. The biology of stress and its resulting discomfort galvanize our efforts to get help and resources we need—care and nourishment to replenish, and support from our friends, families, and communities. They give us the energy and motivation to search ourselves for answers, for meaning, and for strategies to change or make our lives better.

Psychologically, resilience means we successfully command and resolve a trying situation, leading to the learning and confidence we need for next time, leaving us fortified and strengthened for future challenges, perhaps requiring less effort and energy to accomplish what we need when we face a similar challenge.

Stress Resilience Exercise: Let Breath Guide You Home to Your Strength

Most of us forget to breathe when we're stressed or anxious, just when we need our breath's nourishment the most. Let's fix that. I want you to think about a particularly stressful event in your life from the past few weeks. What was going on? How did you feel? How did your body feel? When you were in the midst of the stress, how did you perceive it? Was it good, bad, or somewhere in between? Write this down and tuck it away—we'll get back to it in a bit. This is the first step in a series of exercises we'll be doing throughout this chapter to explore your relationship with stress.

Now take a few deep, cleansing breaths all the way down to your core. Let all of your recall of that stressful experience go. Inhale deeply into your belly and chest to the count of three. Then slowly exhale. Open your mouth. Sigh it out. Soften.

Did you know that one of the first things we do when stressed is to stop breathing deeply? Just when we need the power and solace of our breath to strengthen and activate our center, oxygenate our tissues, and power up our parasympathetic nervous system (to calm and center) it becomes shallow and slow. I see this in my clients frequently as they sit across from me telling their stories of pain, distress, and unease. We all do it. We can unlearn this and use the power of breath to guide us home to our strength.

Physical Stress—Thriving on Challenge

Biologically, all organisms function best when challenged. We're no different. Our bodies, our brains, and our minds learn from each successive challenge, adapting and improving for future challenges. When we get cut or sick from an infection, our immune cells are instantly engaged for healing. They learn and become more robust for next time. Immunological challenge trains our bodies for optimal defensive function, while lack of challenge inevitably leads to loss of function. Living in a sterile or overly clean environment is actually bad for natural immunity—it makes us sicker when we inevitably have to face the outside world.

Scientists call this phenomenon *hormesis*: when environmental challenges to the body improve function. There is an optimal "dose" for every challenge. Deficient *as well as* excessive exposures may be toxic. *Optimal* exposures to challenges, including many toxins, lead to improvements in function.

A common physical challenge that leads to this hormetic effect is movement and physical exertion. Let's take a look in more depth.

The Challenge of Movement and Physical Exertion

Intense forms of movement require high levels of energy to sustain them—this increases oxidative stress, a highly damaging process engendered by ramping up the use of oxygen to make energy. This creates free radicals, highly toxic molecular oxygen species that have the potential to create widespread damage, and can lead to injury, energy loss, and burnout. So why doesn't this fallout of physical exertion kill us?

Consider how on the other end of the spectrum, not moving at all is bad as well. We need the mechanical stress of movement to our muscles and bones. Paralysis leads to bone loss, increased fracture risk, muscle atrophy, and fluid circulation problems. Loss of the highly metabolically active muscle tissue causes energy loss and metabolic disorders. Even excessive sitting has been called "the new smoking," because it reduces longevity as a result of these same factors.

So, what is it that we need?

Balance.

It has been shown that daily, moderate movement, along with short bursts of high intensity exercise, leads to a *decrease* in oxidative stress and its damaging effects despite the production of free radicals. In the face of the challenge of physical exertion, we get better at the cleanup and repair required to manage it as a result of changes in genetic expression. This leads to improvements in energy production and the many benefits of increased strength and endurance. Additionally, the mechanical loading of exercise creates sufficient challenge for our bones and muscles to grow and remain strong, helping to keep us stable and mobile while reducing risk for fracture and muscle injury.

Mind Resilience: Our Brains Need Challenge

It is well known that cognitive engagement is essential for optimizing brain function, intelligence, problem-solving ability, and mental resilience. If we don't use it, we lose it.

Learning is a hugely important way for our brains to engage with challenge. When we learn, we create new connections between brain cells, literally growing the structure and function of our brains. We call this neuroplasticity, the capacity inherent in our brains to grow and change[15]. This is our potential to heal as well as to create bigger better minds.

While learning can be growth fuel for the brain, information overload, as we've already explored in chapter two, leads to toxic distraction, overwhelm, loss of focus, and decrements in learning. Once again, it's all about balance.

THE BIOLOGY OF STRESS: ENERGY

"No mud, no lotus."

—*Thich Nhat Hanh*

So far in this chapter, we've covered a lot of ground. We considered our strong center and equilibrium around that center. We've thought about how to find, protect, nourish, and challenge it. And we've discussed how critical this is as our core is our innermost us.

We've explored some aspects of stress and found that the negative emotion of stress is a construct we can do without—it conflates true stress with what makes us uncomfortable and unhappy. And we've learned how that very discomfort and unhappiness drives positive adaptation to challenge. We found that the right kinds of challenges, in the right amounts, make us grow stronger.

Now we must pull it all together and talk about the actual physiology of stress in order to understand its role as the energy that powers our core. It's critical to understand this so

----

[15] More on neuroplasticity and neural networks in chapter eight, DISCOVER.

we can care for our core, reinforce its energy, and see that it's the source of our ultimate goal: Big Energy. Potential. A healing life.

The Five Core Positive Attributes of Biological Stress

Throughout the remainder of this chapter we'll learn how stress physiology is our functional workhorse. It's what supports our energy as we live and engage with all life's challenges. We'll work with these five core attributes of stress:

1. **How Stress Creates Energy.** The physiology of stress supports all our energy needs, from the continuous background housekeeping functions (think sleep, waking up, and breathing) to the peaks of high intensity action and survival.

2. **How Stress Leads to Learning.** Stress helps us learn and grow into more resilient human beings.

3. **How Our *Perceptions* Calibrate Stress Biology.** Whether we think of stress as good or bad strongly influences whether stress will help or harm us.

4. **How Stress is a *Practice*.** We'll learn to harness the energy of stress to create strong centers for resilience and successful living.

5. **How Self Care Bolsters Stress Biology.** We must support the biology and psychology of stress through all the foundational ways we are learning to care for ourselves.

Balance in the Face of Stress: Allostatic Load

Physically, our survival goals are to maintain function in the face of change. We want to come through the challenges of everyday life alive *and* with all our resources intact for the challenges to come.

In biology this resilience is called allostasis. Allostatic load is the composite of all challenges requiring energy and resources at any given time, including:

- all "housekeeping" functions of the body,

- all movement and action,

- recovery from wear and tear on cells exposed to high metabolic demands.

High allostatic load can lead to loss of critical resources and resilience if recovery is not adequate. Common examples of *high* allostatic load situations are when we're sick, when we're working excessively hard without rest, or when we're persistently sleep deprived. Often these challenges occur at once, amplifying allostatic load and calling on more energy and resources to meet the challenge successfully.

When inadequately supported with energy and resources, a high allostatic load will lead us toward a new balance, which can result in a state of disadvantage and vulnerability for future challenges. In other words, we suffer a loss of resilience. This will occur if we don't know how to support and replenish ourselves with critical resources. Or the challenge of being sick may sap resources that we are unable to completely recover from because of its severity, or because of *preexisting* vulnerabilities—nutrient deficiencies, sleep deprivation, bad habits, unknown genetic predispositions, or inadequate repair and recovery.

Self-Care Supports Resilience by Reducing Allostatic Load

Resilience and allostatic load are where *we* enter the picture—these are the critical points of control over our lives. We have the capacity to decrease our allostatic load (reduce unnecessary stress) and replenish the critical resources we need for next time (build resilience).

First and foremost, we do this through the fundamentals of self-care as described throughout this book. As in all biological systems, there is a minimum threshold for resources needed to energize and organize function optimally.

Through self-care we replenish critical resources needed to support allostatic load: nutrition, sleep, movement, removal of toxins and irritants, and love, for example.

We further improve our resilience by thinking about stress as a positive influence (more on this in a bit). Our old stories about stress being harmful put a damper on how successful we can be at navigating life's challenges. Rising to challenge with a positive and hopeful mindset about the outcome leads to a more supportive stress response, increasing the chances of success.

The Power Players of Stress Biology

Geek alert!

On second thought, no. I was going to say that we're heading into science-y territory as we dive into the biology of stress, and some of you might want to skim or skip. But actually, we're talking about *your* body. These aren't abstract science concepts—this is what's happening inside your body at this very moment. Don't get bogged down by it, but everyone should try to get the gist of it. After all, it's you!

Stress biology is a beautiful and remarkable process, sustaining us through crisis with astonishing precision, as well as supporting us as we breathe, think, move, ponder, get out of harm's way, and climb that mountain. It is a complex, multisystem, finely orchestrated effort that originates in the brain and flows out into the body via nerves, neurochemicals, and hormones, while utilizing nutrients and activating immune cells— all to support our efforts to survive and accomplish what life has put before us.

During our day-to-day lives, stress is part of our standard operation, always making the needed resources available to us for basic function and survival, moment by moment. In its extreme form, stress protects us from excesses of danger, fortifying us for quick response or heroic action.

First Responders: The Electricity of the Autonomic Nervous System (ANS)

When a big challenge presents itself to us, whether it is a brush with danger, a full-on car accident, an intense workout, the emotional shock of upsetting news or catastrophe, or a potentially lethal shift in our physiology (such as low blood sugar or low blood pressure), our automatic nervous system (ANS) kicks in instantaneously without needing our conscious control. As our brain perceives the challenge and potential threat to our survival, within a fraction of a second it triggers the electrical energy of the sympathetic nervous system (SNS), a branch of the ANS. This leads to the immediate outflow of adrenaline to engage and focus our physiology on the urgency.

Most of us are all too familiar with the "adrenaline rush," when adrenaline (also known as epinephrine) released by the SNS concentrates vital resources for survival. Heart rate and strength of heart contraction increase to support blood flow to the brain and muscles.

Respiratory rate goes up to ramp up oxygen availability. Energy is made available instantly in the form of stored glucose or ketones from the liver to fuel the action needed.

The brain becomes one hundred percent focused on the problem at hand. Pupils dilate to let in more light and hearing sharpens. Nonessential functions, such as digestion and reproduction, are suppressed to concentrate energy where it is most needed. Endorphins, testosterone, and dopamine are released, working to mobilize brainpower, motivation, and courage to support productive action and successful resolution of the challenge.

When survival is the issue, these changes in physiology come on strong, eliciting a classic flight, fight, or freeze response. The surge of energy moves us out of harm's way or stops us in our tracks.

As the urgency passes, adrenaline levels decline and the parasympathetic nervous system (PNS) branch of the ANS comes into play. The PNS counteracts the explosive effects of the SNS, shifting us back toward a more relaxed resting state. We can actively harness the calming power of the PNS through meditation, deep breathing, and relaxation strategies to decrease the stimulating effects of stress biology.

Secondary Responders—The Adrenal Glands, Immune Cells, and Neuromodulators

The adrenal glands, immune cells, and neuromodulating hormones show up next to support the first responders, as well as to gently guide us back to equilibrium.

Adrenal Glands

The adrenal glands are also engaged during acute stress, though they take action more slowly than the electricity of the ANS, releasing the hormones cortisol, dehydroepiandrosterone (DHEA), and aldosterone. These support the energy and resources of the stress response, both acutely and long term.

Immune Cells

Immune cells are activated to immediately defend against the effects of trauma and exposure to pathogens and allergens, and to initiate the repair process.

Neuromodulating Hormones

Neuromodulating hormones are also released. Oxytocin is a hormone released by the pituitary gland to augment behavior that mobilizes social support, courage, and motivation to take action on behalf of ourselves and others. Oxytocin is good for the heart, causing vasodilation in the setting of stress, allowing for enhanced blood flow to the heart when demands are greater.

Dopamine, serotonin, and endorphins are neurochemicals released to support motivation, focus, and learning—the brainpower needed for a successful stress response.

Recovery from Acute Stress—Learning

The chemical milieu of the acute stress response sets us up for learning through the process of neuroplasticity. In this way, stress teaches us how to better manage future stress. The attributes of neuroplasticity—to create mind pathways that support future thinking and action—can be purposefully engaged as an intentional "stress inoculation." In this sense we "practice" stress, since with each inoculation, the brain learns and strengthens its performance.

Our own self-reflection about stress is a crucial part of stress recovery that contributes to neuroplasticity and stress resilience. Stress challenges us to discover the meaning in our experiences, and the search for meaning strengthens our ability to face stress successfully in the future. We do this when we review past stressful events or traumas in search of deeper understanding.

Persistent Stress—How the Brain-Thyroid-Adrenal-Mitochondrial (BTAM) Energy Operating System Rises to the Challenge

These are the key players in energy production throughout the body: the brain, the thyroid and adrenal glands, and the subcellular mitochondria. They function to integrate perception, need, and action to support all of our energy requirements. I refer to this harmonic symphony as the brain-thyroid-adrenal-mitochondrial (BTAM) energy operating system, which regulates the energy we need for maintenance and repair and helps drive the pulses of energy required to fuel and sustain us through life's challenges.

This biological system is engaged at all times to create the energy needed to support the basic functions of our bodies. When challenged, the BTAM is amplified in a pulse-like fashion, making available the additional resources and energy we need. In states of chronic stress, the BTAM operating system is our workhorse.

The BTAM Energy Operating System Supports Basic Energy Needs

The BTAM operating system provides the energy for the housekeeping functions of staying alive that do not require our conscious control.

An important example of this is the sleep-wake cycle. Consider what is required of us to wake up in the morning after a night of sleep. Waking up is one of the most physiologically demanding things we do in the course of our daily lives. Our bodies begin to prepare for this strenuous process long before we are consciously awake. Sleep becomes lighter. Our circadian clock within the pineal gland sends information to the hypothalamus about timing for our first awakening. The hypothalamus signals the pituitary gland to release adrenocorticotropic hormone (ACTH), which travels to the adrenal glands, where the adrenal cortex is signaled to produce cortisol, DHEA, and aldosterone. Cortisol is typically at its highest level of the day at the time of awakening, preparing us for the strenuous effort required when going from deep sleep to full awakening, upright posture, and action.

Brain

The brain is constantly monitoring an enormous influx of information about the conditions of our lives, with inputs from all aspects of our internal biology, as well as our minds, emotions, and the environments around us. Our brains rapidly process this information and decisions are made about the level of support needed for energy and resources.

The energy command center within the brain, the hypothalamus, signals the pituitary gland to release its hormones—thyroid stimulating hormone (TSH) and adrenocorticotropic hormone (ACTH)—in both a continuous (maintenance) and pulsing (response to a challenge) fashion. These control hormones communicate directly with the thyroid and adrenal glands, respectively, about the work and energy required by the body to sustain us. When we're challenged, TSH and ACTH levels are ramped up to provide the energy we need.

During persistent states of stress, the hypothalamus also releases the hormone prolactin. With prolonged stress, prolactin decreases production of estrogen and testosterone, leading to reduced fertility, an energy-expensive and nonessential function. It is very common for highly stressed individuals to experience the aftermath of low estrogen and testosterone levels—decreased ovulation, infertility, diminished libido and sexual function, hot flashes, and other symptoms attributable to low sex hormone levels.

It's worth noting that the brain is not picky. It doesn't care what the origin of the stress is. It will mobilize the BTAM energy operating system in very much the same way, just varying intensity levels depending on the need. This means that the trigger for the stress can be external or internal, real or imagined. The myriad emotional and psychological challenges we face can act as triggers to the stress response. Not discriminating, our brains will launch a full-blown stress response to threats that are totally imagined or assumed and the stories we create about our lives.

This is why worrying generates feelings of stress, even though the event has yet to happen. If we imagine catastrophe, our brains will respond to catastrophe, engaging the BTAM energy operating system at a high level. If we imagine courage, strength, and successful outcomes, our brains will respond in kind, and a very different set of responses will be set into play.

Thyroid and Adrenal Glands

The thyroid and adrenals work in concert to mobilize energy. The thyroid gland, which sits at the base of the neck, is like the thermostat in your home. When turned up or down the work accomplished by the HVAC unit will change by regulating the amount of fuel delivered to it and thus converted into usable energy. If the thyroid is the thermostat, the adrenals provide the fuel for the system, making sure there is enough fuel from carbon atoms (derived from glucose, fatty acids, and amino acids) to sustain energy production.

In response to TSH from the pituitary gland, the thyroid gland will produce the hormones thyroxine (T4) and triodothyronine (T3). Thyroid hormones control the amount of work done by the cells by regulating oxygen consumption via changes in genetic expression.

The adrenals, which sit on top of the kidneys, are often referred to as our "stress" glands. The inner parts of the adrenal glands, called the adrenal medulla, make epinephrine (adrenaline) and norepinephrine (noradrenaline) in response to electrical signaling of the ANS during acute stress. While the outer parts of the adrenals, the cortex, make the hormones cortisol, DHEA, and aldosterone, all of which manage the more long-term energy needs of the body.

The job of cortisol is to make sure there are enough carbon atoms available for conversion into chemical energy. Cortisol also helps suppress nonvital biological functions during stress, such as reproduction, digestion, and growth. It helps focus our biological energy on survival and managing the tasks in front of us right now.

DHEA's primary action is related to the brain, priming it for growth and learning, and it ameliorates the potentially harmful effects of cortisol seen in chronic stress. Higher levels of cortisol over time can lead to immune suppression, delayed wound healing, and depression, while higher levels of DHEA moderate these effects, reducing many of the negative effects of chronic stress, lowering our risk for depression, anxiety, inflammation, and neurodegeneration.

Aldosterone maintains blood volume and blood pressure through effects on the kidneys. This action maintains the circulation and transport of the carbon atoms, made available by the action of cortisol, to the vital organs where they will be converted into energy.

Mitochondria

Mitochondria are tiny subcellular organelles, residing within most of our body's cells, which manufacture chemical energy in the form of ATP from carbon atoms, along with oxygen and energy nutrients from food. The delivery of fuel and production of energy within these structures is the common purpose of the BTAM energy operating system.

What Happens When the Demands of Stress Overwhelm the Supply of Resources?

We've met the players of the stress energy operating system. What happens when their ability to respond to persistent challenge (chronic stress) is overwhelmed?

The original teachings about the health effects of stress, derived from the work of Hans Selye and his protégés in the 1950s, were that chronic or persistent stress would lead to a failure in stress adaptation—a breakdown in the components of the stress response, leading to many bad health outcomes. This belief about chronic stress persists to this day.

However, the new science of stress, while standing on the shoulders of these giants, shows us that the stress story is much more nuanced than originally thought. Loss of adaptation to stress is not inevitable. It requires the presence of other vulnerabilities.

There are three primary scenarios in which persistent stress leads to loss of resilience and bad health outcomes:

- When our fundamental beliefs about stress are negative.

- When the requirement for the energy resources needed to power stress outstrips the available reserve.

- When any aspect of the BTAM energy operating system is dysfunctional or has been damaged (as can occur in many illnesses).

Our Beliefs about Stress Determine Resilience

Our minds have powerful effects on our biology. The work of psychologist Alia Crum shows that people who view stress in a positive light—who believe that stress is constructive—are less depressed, more satisfied with their lives, happier, more productive at work, have more energy, and have fewer health problems than those who view stress as negative. Her research shows this effect occurs in spite of the fact that the people with a positive stress mindset are just as stressed and have lives that are just as hard and filled with suffering as their counterparts who have a negative view of stress.

The only difference is that they view stress and its meaning in a more positive light, profoundly improving their long-term health.

Crum's theory to explain these differences is that the positive stress mindset influences how people behave in the face of stress. Rather than avoidance, numbing out, or finding distractions, people with positive stress mindsets tend to walk right into their challenges to face them head on, allowing stress to fuel them as it was designed to. They accept the truth of the challenge before them, plan strategies for tackling it, mobilize resources, and work to discover the meaning in it. They shift the entire stress experience into something that builds resilience through learning, practice, confidence, and improved social support. Through their actions, they create a positive stress experience that further supports their positive understanding of stress, builds resilience, and sets them up for more successful experiences with challenging situations in the future.

For those who believe that stress is bad and leads only to bad things, their mortality rate skyrockets during times of high stress. Their biological stress markers are more dangerous. By contrast, those who perceive stress as fundamentally supportive, have no such increased risk for death. The stress-averse folks have a distinctive physiological response to high stress in which their heart rates go up and the blood vessels feeding the heart constrict at the same time. This coupling of increased demand with decreased blood flow is a set up for disaster, especially in people already primed for heart dysfunction. Those who believe that stress is helpful also experience increases in heart rate as part of a stress response, however, their blood vessels dilate rather than constrict, strengthening and nourishing heart function.

Self-Reflection Exercise: Harness the Positive Energy of Stress

The energy of stress is all about supporting our success. Believe it, claim it, walk right into it. Don't let fear get in your way. Every aspect of the stress response has been designed to

mobilize the energy and resources you need for successful resolution of your challenges.
Practice stepping up to them, even if you are afraid. Let the increased energy of stress
support you.

Can you think of a time when you became overwhelmed or ran away from a stressful
situation? Is it possible to reframe how you understand the feelings of stress in your body?
Could fear and anxiety, though uncomfortable, be perceived in a more positive light, like
getting you out of harm's way and helping you engage with the situation more
powerfully?

How might you have managed your stressful situation differently if you had perceived
the sensations and feelings in your body in a positive way?

Our Reserve of Resources Must Support Stress

I don't have a single client for whom stress isn't a player to some degree in their chronic illness or dysfunction. For many it is overwhelmingly the major issue. They have either been persistent in their efforts to ignore, suppress, or numb the symptoms and messages of stress (how their lives are out of balance), or they have lost biological resilience because of nutritional deficiencies, inadequate sleep and rest, lack of movement, excessive exposure to toxins and irritants, persistent infections or allergies, and are no longer able to support the biological effort of stress. A prolonged and unremitting stress response can cause catastrophic physical and psychological health problems if appropriate action is not taken or if critical resources are lost and not restored.

When stress persists, and if biological resilience is not maintained through self-care, the BTAM energy operating system will eventually show signs of dysfunction through loss of hormonal responsiveness and inadequate energy support to meet continued demands.

The Concept of Adrenal Fatigue

Part of the late phase of chronically unsupported stress is a loss of cortisol production by the adrenals, which can leave us with inadequate levels to support energy needed (by providing optimal carbon fuel sources) for maintenance functions. This will lead to persistent fatigue and poor tolerance to exertion or exercise. Loss of biological energy is a key player in chronic fatigue syndrome and other persistent fatigue states.

The collapse of adrenal function and cortisol levels as the result of persistent stress was described by Hans Selye in the 1950s, in his classic stress model, "the general adaptation syndrome." The loss of adrenal resistance to stress is popularly referred to as "adrenal fatigue," or "adrenal exhaustion." In essence, the adrenals lose *reserve*—the resources they require to sustain hormone levels necessary to make energy and resources available to the body. As a high stress response becomes prolonged, the demands of the body become greater, resources become diminished, and the system, ultimately, cannot sustain itself without replenishment of resources.

In Chinese medicine, adrenal exhaustion is thought of as a loss of foundational life force energy, referred to as "kidney chi deficiency." The goal of acupuncture treatments, Chinese herbs, and lifestyle recommendations is to rekindle this key source of energy. In Functional Medicine, the approach to adrenal fatigue is to unload the adrenals from the excessive demands and challenges put before them (said another way, reduce allostatic load), and to nourish them with self-care through nutrition, sleep, movement, breath, detoxification, and balance.

Modern Western medicine, while beginning to acknowledge the effects of chronic stress on health, does not recognize the critical role of the adrenals and the systems biology of the BTAM energy operating system for maintaining the energy we need to feel well. In this medical model, the adrenals are thought of as either perfectly healthy and functional or failed ("Addison's" disease), not considering the extensive range of function that exists between the two extremes.

Adrenal Fatigue is a Misnomer

However, it is important to understand that the loss of critical energy resources that effect adrenal gland function are also affecting every other aspect of the BTAM energy operating system. In this way, the popular notion of "adrenal fatigue" is a misnomer. The adrenals are never "fatigued" in isolation from the rest of the complex energy operating system. In treating chronic fatigue, it is vital to consider all aspects of the BTAM energy operating system[16]. This integrated, systems biology approach is critical when considering dysfunction with any aspect of the BTAM energy operating system, including the thyroid gland.

Exhaustion Is Purposeful: Take Heed!

Adrenal dysfunction rarely occurs outside the context of global BTAM energy operating system disturbance. In addition, it is not the absolute trajectory of chronically high stress levels. That notion is part of the old stress model that no longer holds up to the scrutiny of science or clinical practice.

In other words, the adrenal glands, as well as all other players in the BTAM energy operating system, can rise to any challenge given an adequate supply of resources to support function, produce energy, and provide protection from potentially noxious effects of the challenges they face.

Said another way: *don't blame the adrenals (or the thyroid or the mitochondria). Instead, heed their message.* Exhaustion and the syndrome of chronic fatigue is an important example of the great wisdom of the body. Fatigue protects us by shutting us down when we are pushed past the point of healthy function. It is the pressure relief valve that flattens us and powers down all but our most vital functions in the face of catastrophe or total overwhelm. It keeps us alive when our reserve is spent. It forces us into laser-sharp consideration of the facts of our dysfunction to mobilize the resources we need.

When we lose resilience in the face of persistent stress or illness, our bodies will eventually bring us to our knees, stopping us, shutting us down, and forcing us to search for meaning and answers. This was my story, as I wrote about in chapter one.

The foundational principle of all of our work to recover from fatigue and to build resilience for the future is to understand that the body is all-wise and always on our side. We're not broken. We just have to decode our bodies' wisdom.

---

[16] See my article series, *Chronic Fatigue Resolution*: karynshanksmd.com/category/5-pillars/chronic-fatigue-resolution/

HEAL KARYN SHANKS MD

BTAM Energy Operating System Dysfunction or Damage

When any aspect of our BTAM energy operating system becomes dysfunctional, or has been damaged, we're at risk for critical energy loss. Dysfunction or damage to the brain and its structures, the thyroid gland, the adrenal glands, and mitochondria can occur as a result of nutrient deficiencies, trauma, infections, toxins, or widespread inflammation from any cause. All these conditions can be discovered and treated. Dysfunction of the hypothalamus, pituitary, thyroid, or adrenals are easy to diagnose and can be resolved with appropriate measures such as nutrients, hormone replacement, and removal of the damaging influences.

Mitochondrial dysfunction can be genetic, though more commonly it results from loss of essential mitochondrial nutrients and the systemic effects of mitochondrial poisons such as drugs, environmental toxins, microbes, and inflammation. These conditions can likewise be readily diagnosed and treated. Persistent fatigue always raises the question of mitochondrial dysfunction. To resolve this, work with a health practitioner who is an expert in Functional Medicine.

Stress Is Our Wise Teacher

The experience of stress is uncomfortable as a way to get our attention. This is the wisdom of our bodies. The discomfort of stress is our opportunity to acknowledge where we are out of balance in our lives, what needs our attention, and how we can create meaningful change. This is our invitation to lean in and listen instead of disconnecting from our body's wisdom. When we ignore the sensations of our bodies, we will always suffer. We must listen deeply. Stress is meant to be our wise teacher.

We can change our relationship to stress. We can understand the process and step into the message. We need to reconsider our commonly held belief that stress is the *source* of our misery. We must claim responsibility for ourselves and for the opportunities that arise in each and every moment for our learning and growth. *Stress is just the messenger, not the challenge or problem itself.* The discomfort of stress is the body telling us that we are ready to engage, with the full force of its resources to back us up, to get us through, and to make us even better for the next time.

We need to reframe or shift our perceptions of stress in the body. Perhaps the physical symptoms of engagement could be experienced as excitement rather than anxiety. If we put a positive spin on it rather than assuming the physical symptoms mean we are in trouble, we can ride the wave of adrenaline and cortisol, capitalize on it with a higher level of effectiveness and exhilaration. This way of responding to our body's cues will improve our lives considerably, making us courageous instead of victimized. We can use the energy of stress to take positive action.

What if we are in over our heads or far out of our comfort zone in an endeavor? Our bodies will tell us. Our charge is to listen carefully. Our bodies will tell us when we've crossed over from engagement to being in trouble. Rather than blaming our bodies or ourselves ("I'm weak," "I'm not capable"), or the external situation ("It's their fault"), we must consider the data being presented to us quite clearly by our bodies and make the necessary adjustments that are being called for (greater effort, better resources, support, or retreat).

If the discomfort of stress becomes chronic, some aspect of our lives is out of balance. It is important to look carefully and consider what our bodies are telling us. The *real* problem isn't with the job, the relationship, or the excessive demands of others. The problem is with how we respond to these challenges. Remember, our bodies are true and clear, while our minds create stories. If our lives are out of balance, our bodies will tell us unequivocally so. Our charge, then, is to claim this domain as our own. To accept full responsibility for it. To take positive action in our lives to create the balance we need. To operate fully from our strong center.

LAST THOUGHTS

We've covered a lot of ground in this chapter. The big takeaways:

- We all have a center that anchors and protects us, which contains the truth and strength of who we are.

- We live in dynamic balance with the world from our center but go with the flow of life.

- We must find, protect, nourish, and challenge our center to keep it strong.

- Stress is the wise messenger, the strengthener, and the physiological energy that powers our center.

In other words, *live* from your center.

Live with abandon, but from the center you've protected and nourished so carefully. Let the risks you take, the projects you tear into, the relationships that test you, the questions you ask, your insatiable curiosity, and your big blazing unstoppable heart—all of it, every bit of your consciously tended, reverently cared for life—let all of it grow your center, grow your soul. Be brave and do all that.

Then pull back. Rest and let go. Protect yourself. Create clear boundaries around your precious self and always be who you are, doing what's best for you in all of it. Accept your suffering: walk straight into it as you breathe into your center, trusting you're up to the challenge. Let it all be messy and imperfect and stressful.

That's a life in balance. That's a life worth living.

Now you're ready for our next lessons in chapter five, RESTORE—We Must Sleep Deeply.

Chapter Five

RESTORE

Sleep Deeply (As well as Rest, Pause, and Play)

As the days grow dark, we grow weary. Retreating to our cozy dens, we lay our heads beneath the stars, and surrender to the solace of deep sleep. Easy as our breath, we pull back and let miracles occur, reappearing with the morning light energized and renewed.

We gift ourselves with pause throughout the day—we breathe, rest, and reset. As we relax and shed our worries, we say "thanks" to ourselves for doing our best, and receive clarity we might not otherwise know about what's next.

We play with wild abandon. Hear us laugh, see us dance, putter, and get lost in our moments.

If we're willing, if we'll allow it, if we set intentions and seek it all—sleep, rest, pause, and play—we emerge strengthened, repaired, and restored.

RESTORATION IS ESSENTIAL TO OUR HEALING LIFE.

Far from passive, the moments and hours we spend sleeping, resting, and playing, are active and dynamic, yielding resources, energy, and pleasure we would not otherwise know. Even so, we live in a culture that condemns us for taking time out. We're taught to burn the candle at both ends—burnout and exhaustion are the badges we earn by doing enough and doing it right.

We know better. And as we stand strong in our truth and courage, we no longer accept this false notion of the successful life as our status quo. We're creating a new, better life.

In chapter two, we *let go*, creating the space we need for healing by removing toxins, irritants, negative energy, and time wasters that get in our way. In letting go we've given ourselves permission for the restoration we require.

When we sleep, we may appear passive, but miracles are happening. When we rest and take pause, we may look unproductive, but we're actively softening and freshening our perspective. And when we play, it may seem as if we're dillydallying and time wasting, but we're creating, growing, and unleashing our genius. With all of our restorative practices we create energy. We expand our minds. We immerse ourselves in the ultimate present moment experiences. We release the excesses of vigilance that kill our creativity and joy. We launch ourselves, each and every night and day—through sleep, breath, pause, and intentional moments—into our potential.

Yes, we must restore. Sleep is the boss. Rest is the necessary pause. Play is the reset that inspires our creative genius.

SLEEP IS THE BOSS

Sleep is powerful medicine. It can't be hacked, passed over, or substituted. There are few aspects of self-care that are as necessary to our healing and energy as good sleep. Sleep is a magical, mysterious time that allows us to power down, repair, replenish, and renew, providing the deepest restoration of energy and wellbeing available to us.

I've seen this countless times in my clients, how the last remaining hurdle to their recovery, the thing that keeps them stuck in fatigue, brain fog, and illness, is not sleeping long enough or not having sleep of sufficient quality to restore them. We *must* sleep. Sleep is the boss.

We all struggle with sleep from time to time. For those of us who have suffered from insomnia, we know the cruel exhaustion and total mind-body devastation that can occur. We also all know the solace resulting from *good* sleep—the clear head, the feeling of lightness, and the enhanced connection to the world around us.

Still, many of us resist sleep, considering it a nuisance that robs us of precious hours of being awake. We get into cycles of staying up late, cutting back on sleep, and using caffeine, sugar, and other stimulants to fuel ourselves during the day. In the end, depriving ourselves of sleep always catches up and slams the brakes on our energy and wellbeing. Sleep is so central to our ability to power up, conserve energy, and repair the damage that has been done while awake, that when we skimp, our bodies will always bring us down (exhaustion, immobility, illness) to survive.

Persistent sleep deprivation leads to exhaustion, burnout, cognitive dysfunction, loss of productivity, mood and behavioral problems, and exacerbation of every conceivable illness. Even mild forms of sleep deprivation are important players in persistent illness, contributing to dysfunction and suffering brought about by excesses of stress, inflammation, chronic infections, toxicity, fatigue, injuries, and mood disorders. Restoring healthy sleep leads to repair and renewal.

Sleep deprivation may be *caused* by illness or critical imbalances that affect the brain's ability to control sleep, or by creating uncomfortable symptoms that make it hard to fall or stay asleep. These include high stress levels, anxiety, trauma, pain, inflammation, or toxicity. Losing the restorative aspects of sleep adds to the burden of illness. In these situations, correcting the underlying cause of the illness leads to recovery of good sleep.

Gretchen

Gretchen was forty-seven years old and suffered from severe insomnia. She was a project manager for a local tech company, worked full time, and was raising three young children with her husband. She'd experienced persistent insomnia twice over a few years, each episode lasting a few months and occurring during times of peak stress. After she became my client, she was able to resolve them with vigilance to good sleep habits, acupuncture treatments, and massage to help relax her. Her sleep was good again.

But then, seemingly out of the blue, she just couldn't stay in a deep sleep. She noted nothing unusual going on in her life at the time. There were no new stresses, her work was good, her family was busy, but they had a good rhythm together. She was generally very happy with her life but simply could not stay asleep. By the end of the day she was exhausted and fell to sleep immediately, but she would then wake up a dozen times or more throughout the night. She felt like she was never getting into a deep sleep and had become physically and emotionally exhausted. She was chronically tired, headachy, irritable, anxious, and could not stay focused at work. She was using caffeine to stay alert and awake during the day.

When she came to see me again, she had already been to her acupuncturist and was getting massages. She was eating well, exercising regularly, and was keeping up with her meditation and journaling practice. She was doing all the "right" things, the same habits and practices that had been keeping her feeling well and balanced for years. But it was becoming increasingly difficult to keep up with her self-care due to fatigue.

Although a physical exam and blood work were normal, clearly something was wrong. As we talked, she noted that her menstrual cycles were a bit longer, she had skipped a couple of periods, and she was hot and sweaty many nights. She also noticed that she was losing more hair, was having trouble remembering things, and her skin seemed drier. All these are symptoms of decreased estrogen—which, if sufficiently lowered, can also interfere with sleep. The brain is rich with estrogen receptors and even subtle changes in estrogen levels in the blood can have profound effects for many women. At her age, it was the biology of life. She was moving to a new equilibrium, but one that didn't work for her. Her self-care and regimen of relaxation modalities and healthy living were great, but not enough to offset the effects of low estrogen. Fortunately, we could help her reestablish her old sleep balance.

We took measures to improve her estrogen equilibrium, including use of a low-dose estrogen patch. I spoke with her one week later, and she was ecstatic to report that by the second night after putting on the patch her sleep had improved, and by the one-week point she was sleeping through the night and feeling more rested in the morning. She felt like a new woman. Her mood and energy improved substantially. Several years out, while continuing hormone therapy, her sleep remained excellent, her energy robust, her mind stayed clear, and she felt wonderful.

For Gretchen, menopausal hormone imbalance was an important cause of her insomnia. Correcting the underlying imbalance led to restoration of good sleep. Now, let's consider the opposite, a case where not sleeping *led* to illness.

Tom

Tom was the walking wounded. He felt terrible. He came to see me after several years of depression, lethargy, and poor exercise tolerance. He had body aches and joint pain. His head felt fuzzy and he had trouble concentrating. He tried to keep up with his exercise but found it unusually grueling and exhausting. He was eating the standard American diet with lots of processed grains, sugar, dairy, and fast food. He felt trapped in a job that he did not like but didn't feel he could risk making a change and still provide for his family. He was having trouble controlling his irritability around his family and was easy to anger. He was feeling lost and out of control. And he only slept five to six hours each night.

In situations like Tom's, our Functional Medicine approach is to get at root causes—those things that support us, fuel us, and get at what we're made of. So, one of the first things we did was have him start a nutrient-dense, low inflammation potential diet (the FINE food plan detailed in chapter seven), and we corrected several nutrient deficiencies through food and high quality supplements. By adhering to the food plan, he felt considerably better and became hopeful about eventual full recovery.

But Tom continued to stay up late and rise early to get his workouts in before taking the kids to school and starting his own workday. This was a long-standing pattern, and he thought it worked. But it was such a routine part of his day that he did not recognize he was still sleep deprived. Yes, he might have been fifty percent better, but he wanted more. So, as we talked, I convinced him to gradually move his bedtime to an earlier hour, to remove all electronics from his bedroom and always use blue light filters when using them and stop at least two hours before lights-out. I also suggested that he try to get outside at mid-day to receive natural light for at least thirty minutes to help reset his circadian rhythm.

He worked on this for a while and gradually got his bedtime moved up to 10:00 p.m. (it had been 12:00 to 1:00 a.m.), which allowed him to get sufficient sleep before getting up at 5:45 a.m. to work with his trainer. Along with sustaining his food plan, he now felt one hundred percent better! Just like his normal self. His energy was high, focus and concentration good, and his mood happy and stable. His exercise tolerance improved greatly. He falls off the wagon from time to time, as old habits can die hard, but he now knows the power of good sleep habits in his life.

WHAT MAKES SLEEP SO IMPORTANT

We can all relate to the solace and deep comfort of a good, long night's sleep and the many ways it makes us feel rejuvenated. But we sometimes take for granted *why* it makes us feel so much better. While sleep is complex, there are four foundational functions of sleep that lead to its profound restorative properties:

- energy conservation and renewal,

- detoxification and cleansing of the brain,

- circadian rhythm regulation of physiology, and

- memory consolidation and dreaming.

Energy Conservation and Renewal

Being awake is energy expensive, regardless of our level of activity. We are not built to sustain a high level of energy use without built-in breaks. Sleeping overnight allows for our body to power down—body temperature drops, and our body systems are less active. Blood pressure and heart rate go down and our digestive system rests. The body goes into a deep state of quiet, reducing energy stress on our bodies, restoring us for the next day of wakefulness.

The energy conservation aspect of sleep is facilitated by the brainstem—the lower part of the brain, which makes us feel sleepy, urging us to sleep after a period of wakefulness. This neurological action is supported by production of the brain-calming hormone melatonin, produced by the pineal gland in response to light reduction and darkness (meditation also stimulates melatonin production). These powerful factors make it hard for us to resist surrendering to sleep.

Sleep also supports our daily renewal of fresh energy. Energy renewal depends on an integration of many vital functions. The powering down of energy conservation we just talked about, as well as the antioxidant, detoxification, hormonal, and repair aspects of sleep all contribute to our ability to make optimal energy when we're awake.

For example, persistent sleep deprivation will result in loss of circadian control of adrenal hormone secretion. Recall that our morning levels of the adrenal hormone, cortisol, should be at their highest of the day to support the physiological challenge of waking up. If we lose this circadian control of cortisol and levels fall off, we're left with suboptimal fuel to support our energy needs.

Persistent Sleep Loss Causes Weight Gain

The loss of energy resilience that comes with persistent sleep loss leads to increased appetite and food consumption to compensate for the loss of fuel for energy. As a result, weight gain is a common manifestation of persistent sleep deprivation. Interestingly, sleep deprivation and circadian rhythm disruption can lead to weight gain independent of calorie consumption. Even without eating more, the altered hormonal control leads to weight gain. Thus, in overweight people who are not sleeping well, it is important to correct sleep patterns to reestablish normal hormonal control before changing diet. This will release an important block to normal metabolism and achieving ideal body weight. By correcting sleep problems without restricting calories, most people will lose body fat.

Detoxification and Cleansing of the Brain

Antioxidant protection and the removal of neurotoxic waste products are some of the most important restorative functions of sleep. The energy expensiveness of being awake leads to the accumulation of toxic debris from the chemistry of energy production—the price we must pay for using oxygen to make energy. This toxicity, referred to as *oxidative stress*, must be neutralized and removed to keep our cells and tissues healthy. Our cells depend on protection from dietary as well as intrinsic antioxidants, such as melatonin.

We literally cleanse our brains while we sleep. The spaces between cells throughout the body play a dynamic role in clearing toxins and debris. Within the brain this is accomplished by cerebral spinal fluid (CSF) that fills those spaces between cells. Research shows that when we sleep our brains shrink. Studies done on mice demonstrate brain shrinkage by as much as sixty percent. This allows for increased flow of the CSF around the brain and through every fold and crevice, allowing the fluid to sweep away the toxic debris that accumulates while we're awake. This includes proteins such as beta-amyloid, toxic components of the destructive brain plaques observed in the brains of people who've died from Alzheimer's disease.

HEAL KARYN SHANKS MD

If we don't sleep, not only does the additional wakefulness demand energy to sustain it—adding to the pool of toxic oxidative stress—but our brains can't clean things up. The toxins, debris, and waste products accumulate around the brain with nowhere to go. Therefore, it is not at all surprising that a strong link exists between sleep deprivation and risk for dementia and neurodegenerative disorders, including Alzheimer's, all linked to brain toxicity.

Circadian Rhythm Regulation of Physiology

The circadian rhythm of light and dark guides a multitude of body functions autonomously through the solar cycle. Not only is our sleep pattern affected by our circadian rhythm, but our circadian rhythm is, in turn, affected by our sleep.

Sleep, as a biological function, has evolved with the changing, rhythmic aspects of our earth—the solar, lunar, and seasonal cycles. This relationship has become part of our foundational genetic wiring and optimal sleep stays true to these cycles.

The light-dark solar cycles, seasons, lunar cycles, and temperature fluctuations of the earth have become ingrained in our genetics and biology—we are wired to live according to the dictates of these environmental cycles. When we get out of sync, our health can suffer. While many of our modern technological advances allow us to subvert the pressures of nature's fluctuating conditions—like electricity, artificial light, and electronic devices—our best health, energy, and wellbeing occur when we live according to nature's rhythms, sleeping when it's dark and being awake when it's light. Light produced by electricity and electronic devices interferes with healthy sleep by altering our internal circadian rhythm and control of sleep physiology.

Our internal sleep-wake cycles adhere closely to the light-dark cycle of the sun—in fact our biology is entrained at the molecular level to use light and dark signals to control sleep and regulate key aspects of our biological function. This is accomplished by turning on and off specialized genes in our DNA known as "clock genes." Clock genes express themselves according to the relative amount of light transmitted to the brain and form the basis of our circadian rhythm.

Clock genes exert control over the many rhythmic aspects of our internal biology, such as sleep and rest, wakefulness and activity, body temperature, blood pressure, hormone secretion, energy production, and detoxification. Clock gene expression has been exquisitely attuned over the millennia in response to eons of experiences. There is an optimal expression (and therefore optimal function) of these genes throughout the day; however, they will respond to whatever environment they find themselves in to help maintain equilibrium.

For our clock genes to exert positive control over our physiology, it is best for us to sleep at night, when it's dark, and be awake during the day, with regular and adequate natural light exposure. It is ideal to receive a minimum of an hour of outdoor light exposure each day—preferably at noon when the sun is closest to the earth—and adhere to sleep patterns that have us awake when it's light and asleep when it's dark.

Darkness favors physiology that allows for sleep, critical energy preservation and repletion, and for the core physiological functions that restore, cleanse, and revitalize us. Light favors a physiology that coordinates the higher energy functions of the body. Thus, it is no surprise that light deprivation, as well as sleep deprivation, interferes with all key hubs of our internal biology. This leads to myriad health problems, including elevated blood pressure, digestive and gut motility problems, hormone imbalances (including PMS, menopausal symptoms, and infertility), weight gain, increased inflammation, increased susceptibility to infectious disease, cognitive dysfunction, and dementia.

Memory Consolidation and Dreaming

Sleep is critical for editing and interpreting all the information collected by our brains while awake. Sleep reinforces memory in all stages of sleep, but primarily early in the sleep cycle. It has been suggested that sleep should be delayed for six to eight hours following traumatic events to allow sufficient time for the waking brain to work through or resolve the trauma before the sleeping brain consolidates the raw experiences into long-term memories. By contrast, sleep deprivation interferes with the creation of new memories, which may lead to cognitive impairment.

Dreams occur during the rapid eye movement (REM) stages of sleep. (More about the stages of sleep follows later in this chapter.) The brain is highly active during this time, while the muscles of the body (except for eyes, ears, heart, and diaphragm) are paralyzed. This may be the only time the mind activates outside the bounds of our conscious control.

Dreamtime is thought to be when our untethered brains are the most intelligent, insightful, and creative, potentially leading to innovation, discovery, and freethinking. The purpose of dreams is controversial, but Carl Jung, the venerable late psychoanalyst who wrote extensively about dream theory, hypothesized that dreams carry symbolic content from the unconscious as a means to bring important wisdom into our awareness.

WHAT GETS IN THE WAY OF GOOD SLEEP?

We know how wonderful a good night's sleep feels, how it unleashes our feeling of potential for the day before us. We also know how miserable a bad night's sleep makes us feel, and now we understand some of the biological effects of poor sleep. So why are so many of us choosing to forego optimal sleep? Why do we skimp here when doing so clearly hijacks our best function and happiness? Good sleep is within our control.

Common Reasons for Not Getting Enough Sleep

We've developed bad habits that rob us of the restorative sleep we need to stay well. Intentional sleep debt is the number one cause for our culture's epidemic of sleep loss. The excessive stresses of modern living can leave us feeling tired, but wired, and unable to fall or stay asleep. Or perhaps we're worriers and our thoughts and concerns about tomorrow are keeping us up.

Our sleep environments can interfere with good sleep due to noise, light, or discomfort. We may have infants or small children living in our homes. Uncomfortable bedding can be an annoyance. And excessive exposure to daytime light, especially blue light emitted from electronic screens, will keep us up by reducing our melatonin production. Even small amounts of light (a single photon!) emitted into your sleep environment causes a decrease in melatonin production, the hormone responsible for calming the brain in preparation for sleep.

Acute and persistent mood problems such as anxiety, depression, and bipolar disorder can also interfere with both quantity and quality of sleep. And a host of health problems will interrupt sleep: hormone imbalances, body pain and discomfort, urinary tract dysfunction, primary sleep disorders such as sleep apnea and movement disorders (periodic limb movement disorder, also known as restless legs syndrome, is common), circadian rhythm disturbances, chronic infections, allergies, inflammation, gastrointestinal disorders, and blood sugar instability.

Some of these reasons for not being able to sleep well are, themselves, the very result of sleep deprivation. It can become a vicious cycle. When we're deprived of needed sleep, a wide range of health problems can occur, which themselves contribute to not sleeping well.

The most obvious effect of insufficient sleep is tiredness—the result of physiological energy debt. This, by itself, results in reduced effort, motivation, desire, and performance—some of the very attributes that many of us feel most define us as individuals.

Many of the common problems associated with the vicious cycle of sleep deprivation are the result of the persistent activation and acceleration of our body's stress system. (Remember the BTAM energy activation system from chapter four?) We must use this system to fuel the higher demands placed upon us by sleep deprivation. However, as we've discussed before, there's a price to pay for this. Persistently elevated activation of the BTAM energy activation system leads to depletion of critical resources, loss of resilience, and undesired alterations in our physiology that lead to myriad problems: fatigue, increased feelings of stress, loss of emotional resilience, mood problems (depression, anxiety, irritability), increased inflammation, increased appetite and weight gain, digestive and gut motility dysfunction, loss of cognitive function, loss of competence and performance in tasks, increased susceptibility to accidents and mistakes, increased sensitivity to pain and discomfort, and hormone imbalance problems (cortisol, estrogen, testosterone, melatonin).

WHAT CONSTITUTES GOOD SLEEP?

We understand why sleep is important. We know some of the toxic consequences of lack of sleep and how they rob us of ourselves. We've seen some of the most common causes of lack of sleep. But how do you know if you're one of the many sufferers of sleep deprivation? As with Tom in the earlier story, it may not be immediately apparent. What does it mean to sleep well? The answer will vary from one individual to the next. The specifics—number of hours needed, best particular time of night for sleeping, or waking time, for instance—are unique to each of us. But based on what we've discussed up to this point, you can ask yourself four simple questions when evaluating your sleep:

- Is it sustained long enough to meet your unique needs?

- Is it deep enough and uninterrupted?

- Does it align with the solar cycle of light and dark?

- Are you waking up feeling refreshed and restored?

Is Sleep Sustained Long Enough to Meet Your Unique Needs?

It is important that we sleep *long enough* to meet our needs. We are all unique in what those needs are, and they change with age, level of activity, and energy requirements. They've changed as we've moved from living according to the natural conditions of the earth and her light-dark cycles, to using artificial light. Our ancestors slept many more hours, on average, than we do today.

Sleep research is tricky because it's hard to quantify optimal sleep time in a world that is so changed by the usual triggers and mediators of sleep—exposures to light and dark, and a multitude of lifestyle characteristics. These are factors that are difficult to control even in a research setting. However, a gross approximation of optimal sleep times are as follows: Newborns sleep most of the time—on average fourteen to seventeen hours per day. Then, the need for sleep gradually decreases as we age. Teens require eight to ten hours on average, young adults seven to nine hours, and adults ages twenty-six to sixty-four need an average of seven to nine hours of sleep per night. Older adults need seven to eight hours on average. For people who are severely fatigued, ill, or highly active, longer periods of sleep are necessary.

These are all averages determined from observation of modern people sleeping spontaneously in conditions in which we've overridden the natural light-dark cycles with artificial light sources. Many experts hypothesize that our sleep needs are actually much greater than these, and that we sleep longer and better with more daytime exposure to natural light and decreased exposure to artificial light (especially the blue light emitted from electronic devices, which inhibits melatonin production) at night.

I ask all of my clients to evaluate their personal optimal sleep needs. They do this by observing the amount of sleep they actually get when it's unscheduled, by going to bed at a time of their choice and getting up naturally without an alarm, all after a day with at least an hour of outdoor light exposure, movement, and healthy eating. In my experience, folks' assessment of "optimal" sleep (as opposed to "sufficient" sleep) is always more than the experts predict. My own observations about myself are that I need nine to ten hours of uninterrupted sleep every night to feel my absolute best.

Is Sleep Deep Enough and Uninterrupted?

The quality of our sleep is as important as the amount of time we spend in bed. This means we must pass through the structural attributes of sleep that we refer to as the sleep stages. We don't yet understand all the details about sleep stages and the roles they play in the restorative functions of sleep, but we do know that they are necessary.

As we move through a full night of sleep, we cycle through all four non-rapid eye movement (NREM) stages as well as rapid eye movement (REM) sleep. We spend approximately eighty percent of our time in stages one through four NREM sleep, each defined by the particular types of brain waves that occur and our potential for arousal. Each of the sleep stages has unique brain wave patterns as well as eye and muscle movement characteristics. We begin in stage one, rapidly advance to stage two, and end up in the deeper, coma-like stages three and four. Brain waves become slower, and it becomes increasingly difficult to arouse. These deeper stages of sleep are necessary for many of the restorative actions of sleep that we've talked about.

The remaining twenty percent of our sleep time is spent in REM sleep. REM cycles are typified by chaotic brain wave activity, muscle paralysis, and burst of rapid eye movement. This is the time when we dream. As we progress through the night, REM sleep periods increase in length while deep sleep decreases. Our most vivid dream recall occurs when we are aroused out of REM sleep.

If we become unable to spend enough time in the deeper stages of sleep due to interruptions or conditions that awaken us—such as pain, abnormal movement, physiological imbalances such as inflammation or hormone deficiency, or environmental disruptions—those deep restorative phases of sleep do not occur. This results in nonrestorative sleep, experienced as fatigue and, when persistent, with the impairments and illnesses we've reviewed.

Does Sleep Align with the Solar Cycles of Light and Dark?

We've already discussed the importance of aligning sleep with our natural circadian rhythms, but I want to underscore that the literature on circadian rhythm disruption and health is huge. We're designed to take in large amounts of natural light during the day, so much so that normal physiological function depends on it. Low daytime light exposure, such as occurs when we stay inside all day, is associated with many problems involving energy, mood, sleep, hormone balance, and weight control.

Sleeping in the dark and experiencing reduced light in the evening—as our ancestors did, before our extensive use of artificial light—downshifts levels of stress hormones and inflammation mediators, and improves sleep quality. Shift workers who are awake during the night and sleep during the day, completely losing the influence of light-dark solar cycles on their bodies, have a reduced lifespan and increased risks for a myriad of health conditions.

Are You Waking Up Feeling Refreshed and Restored?

This is by far the most important question of all. Feeling refreshed and restored is the best indicator of whether we have received sufficient high quality sleep. We don't need fancy tests to figure this out. Our bodies know.

How do you know? Each of the four sleep cycle categories overlaps and can be difficult to separate out, but if you are at all uncertain about the quality of your sleep, or have difficulty reading the signals of your body, observe yourself carefully and answer these questions:

- Are you less alert and awake than you would like to be?

- Are your motivation, effort, and performance of tasks not where you want them to be?

- Are others expressing concern about your performance?

- Are you yawning, irritable, restless, having headaches, or falling asleep at inappropriate times during the day?

- Do you snore or wake up startled in the night?

- Do you need to wake up to an alarm in the morning?

- Do you depend on caffeinated drinks, stimulants, or sugar to get through the day?

If you answered "yes" to any of these questions, you may not be getting enough sleep, or sleep of sufficient quality. I've had clients who spend ample time in bed, and think they are sleeping, but we discover problems that interfere with their ability to stay in the necessary deep stages of sleep (such as sleep apnea or periodic limb movement disorder). Treating these problems resolves their fatigue.

HOW TO RESTORE HEALTHY SLEEP

Ask for Help

As we saw, there are many health conditions that can make sleep difficult. It is important to work with a trusted health practitioner to get these problems solved.

You may need lab tests to check for thyroid and adrenal function, nutrient levels, iron stores, and indicators of inflammation.

You may need to have a sleep study—a home overnight oximetry test or a more extensive test performed at a professional sleep lab. In the latter, specialists monitor the quality of your sleep, oxygen levels, movements that may lead to arousals from sleep, quality of your breathing, and in some cases, brain wave activity. I order sleep studies routinely for my clients who have persistent fatigue without an obvious cause after a thorough evaluation, or if they had symptoms suggestive of a sleep disorder, such as sleep apnea or periodic limb movement (PLM). PLM leads to arousals out of the deeper stages of sleep, decreasing the restorative aspects of sleep. Sleep apnea—inappropriate pauses in breathing during sleep caused by airway obstruction or brain dysfunction—leads to oxygen deprivation as well as frequent arousals, diminishing sleep quality and impairing brain function.

Make Good Sleep a Practice

When we were kids, sleep came so easily. We didn't have to think about it. But life gets complicated, and we have to turn to intentional commonsense practices to make good sleep happen. We've got to have a plan and make space for it in our lives. We've got to make sleep one of our core self-care habits.

We know sleep is the boss. Nothing turns us around faster than beautiful sleep.

Plan a regular bedtime that makes sense for your life and stick to it. The brain likes habitual behavior, sets up neural pathways, and will get into the groove. Your clock genes will adjust to support you.

Plan for *enough* sleep. Stay in bed long enough to meet your unique sleep needs. This will be different for everyone.

If you experience tiredness or lack of restoration after a night of sleep, you're either not getting enough or the quality of sleep is lacking. If you are recovering from an illness, you'll need more sleep than usual.

Prepare Your Body for Sleep

Eat well.

A richly nutritious diet leads to a healthier body and brain, and establishes the foundational biology for good sleep. We will cover what kind of diet to eat in the next chapter, but no matter what, eat lightly at night, not within two hours of going to bed, and fast (no food—water only) for twelve to fourteen hours overnight from the time of your last meal. Make sure you're getting enough protein. Avoid all commercial animal products, which are high in proinflammatory fats that can disrupt sleep. Don't rush eating—this impairs digestion, a common sleep disruptor.

Create a healthy microbiome.

Our gut microbiome—the communities of bacteria and other microbes that reside within our intestines and support health—affect our sleep, and our sleep, in turn, affects the microbiome. Gut microbes influence our sleep patterns through their effect on clock genes—potentially impacting hormone balance, energy metabolism, detoxification, immune regulation, and circadian rhythm. When we don't sleep well, our microbiome is disrupted due to negative effects of stress hormones, low energy, and oxidative stress, creating a vicious cycle of dysfunction. We'll talk more about your microbiome in chapter seven.

Morning jumpstart.

Start each day with something hot to drink like pure water, tea, or bone broth (save coffee, if allowed on your food plan, for later in the morning, when cortisol levels are dropping naturally—it will be more effective). This wakes up the gut and signals the body that a new day is beginning. Rest a bit while consuming rather than leaping right out of bed and into action. As we've discussed, the process of waking up is the most stressful event of the day physiologically. This is a good time to meditate, write in your journal, or review affirmations that set a positive tone to start your day.

Boost natural light exposure during the day and allow darkness to set in at night.

Spend time outdoors or near windows. When possible, an hour of sunlight at noon every day is best. Then avoid excesses of light and electronics for at least a couple of hours before bedtime. This allows for your brain's circadian rhythm to get in sync, optimizing clock gene expression and releasing melatonin to calm your nervous system, preparing for deep sleep.

Use blue light filters on your electronic screens or glasses and read on devices with a black background (or read paper books!). Sleep in the dark—use blackout shades and remove all sources of light, such as phones, clocks, and all electronic devices. Remove all mirrors, which can amplify light, from your sleeping spaces. Even small amounts of light will inhibit melatonin production, a key driver of sleep.

Remove electromagnetic field (EMF) sources.

While inadequately studied to date, there is an abundance of anecdotal evidence that EMF may be disruptive to sleep via its effects on electrical communication within the body. It is hypothesized that EMF exposure would especially affect the brain and nervous system—the main control centers for sleep. To optimize sleep, experiment with removing all electronic devices, cordless phone bases, and turn off the wireless communication networks within your home during sleep.

Stay well hydrated throughout the day.

Drink ample fluids—a minimum of two to three quarts per day for most people. However, avoid drinking too close to bedtime or your full bladder may awaken you during the night. Hold off on fluids for at least two hours before going to sleep.

Move and exercise your body every day.

Movement throughout the day supports a healthy body and brain and helps moderate excesses of stress. Intense exercise early in the day helps with deeper sleep, but avoid it late in the day as the increase in stress hormones can interfere with falling to sleep.

Limit caffeine use to early-mid-morning.

Caffeine helps override the perception of tiredness from sleep deprivation by its effect on adenosine receptors (adenosine is the brain chemical responsible for making us feel sleepy). But its stimulant effects, effects on stress hormone secretion, and delay of melatonin secretion from the pineal gland can interfere with sleep, even many hours later.

Consider the half-life of caffeine. The half-life of any drug is the time it takes the body to clear out half of the dose ingested. Said another way, at one half-life of the drug, half of the dose remains. Caffeine has a half-life of five to six hours, so if you take your morning coffee at 10 a.m., you'll still have half that dose in your body at 3 p.m,. and a quarter of that dose at 8 p.m., the time of day when most of us are winding down. Imagine if you take a cup of coffee at 3 p.m,. you still have half that amount of caffeine on board at bedtime. So, yes, your morning cup of coffee, regardless of when it is consumed, will affect you at bedtime.

Avoid excesses of alcohol.

Any quantity of alcohol can impair sleep. Some folks are very sensitive to this effect and should avoid it all together.

Prepare Your Mind for Sleep

Let go of the day.

Start the process of letting go of the concerns of your day at least two to three hours before laying your head on your pillow. Again, you should turn down lights and turn off electronics. Decrease noise and begin to move into the more restful phase of your day.

Unload your worries and to-do list onto your peripheral brain (write them down or enter them into your electronic device). This will allow you to rest rather than worry about what needs to be done tomorrow.

Allow yourself to relax. This is especially beneficial for those stressful days when your mind is not quite ready to settle down. This practice could be as simple as reading an enjoyable book before bed, doing a calming meditation, a guided meditation, quiet prayer, listening to soothing music, or other settling, calming activity. Some meditations are energizing and may not be conducive to letting go into a deep sleep—trust your body to tell you what works best for you.

Meditate during the day. Daytime meditation, practiced in the morning or as late as early evening, balances the stress and nervous systems, making sleep more available to us at the end of the day. Meditation increases the production of melatonin from the pineal gland and creates a biochemical milieu that favors deep sleep.

If you have a hard time getting your mind to quiet down at bedtime, use affirmations about deep sleep that activate the power of your intentions:

I let go, rest my mind and sleep deeply.

Thank you for the perfect sleep and restoration.

I am safe and comfortable in my bed.

Create an Environment That Supports Good Sleep

Assess your bedding. Are your mattress, pillows, and covers perfectly comfortable? Are you warm or cool enough?

Work to remove all clutter from your bedroom. Those piles of clothes, books, or work-related stuff stress us, even when we're not aware of them, keeping us from the deep letting go we need to sleep well.

Use Safe Sleep Aids to Support Your Sleep

Work with herbs that can calm the brain and assist with sleep: chamomile, lemon balm, valerian, kava, skullcap, passionflower. These come in combination formulas that are safe and affordable. Note that there are some people who experience paradoxical alertness when using valerian.

Try safe nutritional supplements to relax the brain: GABA, 5-HTP, l-theanine, magnesium glycinate, glycine. Follow manufactures' guidelines or the advice of your trusted health practitioner.

Melatonin can help reestablish the internal circadian rhythm that helps regulate sleep. It can be especially helpful for time zone changes, shift workers, sleep changes associated with aging, and inflammation. Start with one to three mg taken in the evening, an hour or two prior to bedtime.

For those who are exhausted from too much stress, but too wired to sleep, adrenal supportive nutrients and herbs may be helpful. Phosphatidyl serine taken at bedtime is an excellent neutralizer of the stimulating effects of cortisol on the brain. Work with a trusted healthcare provider who is knowledgeable about such treatments.

Therapeutic modalities such as massage, acupuncture, energy medicine, or hypnotherapy can be very helpful for sleep.

Manage Complex Sleep Disorders

Your sleep may be particularly challenged by pain and discomfort, menopausal symptoms, or other distressing symptoms. Work with a trusted health practitioner on these problems.

You may have restless legs or sleep apnea. Your current symptoms may make this obvious. A sleep study and work with your doctor will help sort this out.

Some people need sleep medication as a "bridge," allowing them to sleep as part of their recovery plan, while the other aspects of their illness are being addressed. The need to correct sleep problems with the use of medications must be balanced with their addictive potential, habit-forming nature, and tendency to disrupt normal sleep architecture. Work with a pro.

Remember: there is always a solution. Mobilize your health support team. Get a new opinion if necessary.

Exercise: Create a Personal Sleep Plan

Work with the following questions to help you create your initial sleep goals and a plan for better, more restorative sleep. Take a moment to write these down. Remember, keep this simple and doable. Start with just three small things to work on.

Name Your Personal Sleep Goals

What do you want to accomplish? Have more energy? Feel less tired? Have more enthusiasm and vitality for the day? Feel more like yourself? Name them and write them down.

Then, Name the Three Things You Most Need to Work on to Improve Your Sleep

Based on what you've read so far, contemplate what you need in your own life to achieve the sleep goals you just names. How can you sleep better? Choose an earlier bedtime? Make your bedroom darker? Set aside more time for relaxation before bed? Decrease your daytime caffeine intake?

Use the power of three here. Create your list of three things to start your journey to improved sleep:

1.

2.

3.

First Action Steps toward Better Sleep and Increased Vitality

Again, using the power of three, list the three action steps you will take tonight to improve your sleep:

1.

2.

3.

BEYOND SLEEP— REST, PAUSE, AND PLAY

To restore we've got to sleep, but it's also essential for us to unplug throughout the day. Taking necessary pauses helps us reset, reinvigorate, and carve out space to both rest and move consciously through our days. But, like sleep, we've forgotten how to pause—to rest, unplug, and play.

As we've seen, sleep can be hard. But, rest? That's *really* hard! And play? How do we do that again? Well-practiced achievers, shouldered with the responsibilities of life, many of us leave little space for downtime or fun. To unplug is to be left behind, or makes us guilty, selfish, and lazy. Or maybe we're just plain stuck—we really, really want to, but we don't remember *how* to pause or play.

How did we forget? Wasn't that second nature to us as children? Weren't we busy, purposeful, and engaged every waking moment with our own spontaneous agenda? Weren't we free, creative, and exploding with curiosity, experimentation, and growth? And then we dropped in little heaps right where we were, letting it all ago, without care or worry, to take our needed rest. Never overthinking or judging, just claiming what we needed. How did we morph from little mad, spontaneous geniuses into overworked, regimented, exhausted adults?

We've got to pay the rent and take care of our families, but to find Big Energy and potential, we must also reclaim the inner mad geniuses we've lost—who flow, who are free, who live with abandon right now, and who take pause as they need it, without judgment or fear.

What Do Necessary Pauses Look Like?

Total Shut Down

Our necessary pause may be taking a nap—total shut down of our conscious mind. Or grabbing a break to stare off into space, releasing focused engagement with our life tasks. But just because we are still doesn't mean we are passive. These periods of stillness fill us with the restorative energy we need to carry on and be our best. Yes, sometimes we've just got to drop and let go.

Active Pauses

Necessary pauses may also be quite active. These activities shift us out of our routine and ordinary time. Breaks from hard work and deep focus, to a larger, softer perspective and deeper awareness. This is hard. This takes guts. But we need it so badly.

Believe it or not, there's time. We have seconds for a single conscious breath or two. Breaths that shift our attention, however briefly, into present-moment awareness. Breath that creates space between our thoughts and our next actions. Pauses that invite inspiration, insights, great ideas, or solutions to our problems. Or that simply refresh and renew.

On busy days at work, I depend on such precious pauses. I step away from my desk, walk to the window, look out over the trees and grass, and breathe deeply, taking it all in as I release my previous thoughts and activities. Sometimes I take sojourns to the sink to slowly wash my hands, allowing the sensation of cool water and lavender soap engage my awareness, ritually shifting my focus away from my last client, preparing me for the next. All in a matter of seconds.

Keep in mind that it's best not to take on too much too quickly. Plan your pauses in advance and keep them to no more than three as you're getting used to this. Perhaps set a timer to remind you when it's time to pause—even the thirty-second pauses can be hard to remember in the midst of a busy day!

Play

Play can be most anything we do for sheer enjoyment. I play when I write sometimes. Play can have rules and structure, and can call on our skills and accomplishments, but most importantly, it's fun. We pretend, imagine, or improvise. We get lost in something we're good at. We become completely focused in the moment of high competition. We flow. There may be time limits, but the process is time expanded—we're not aware of time. In play, we're fully engaged in the moment.

Puttering

Necessary pauses may also be in how we allow time for putter, a type of play. Puttering is action with a purpose, but without limitation of time, sequence, or endpoint. We can putter at most anything, from fixing things in the workshop, to rearranging furniture, decorating a room, or sorting through closets. Done without time stress, puttering releases us from ordinary time—our regretful, worried, and busy minds—and brings us back to present-time awareness.

Puttering actively engages us with tasks and movements that may be quite specific, structured, and productive. But what makes puttering distinct from work, is how it releases us from the constraints and pressures of time, expectations, and productivity that drain our energy. We're rejuvenated through the joy and satisfaction of our accomplishments.

Puttering can be the key to finding solutions to our problems. We set the problem aside, enter the present-moment awareness of our project and ideas flood in while we're not actively searching for them. Puttering gets us out of our own way.

Laughter

Laughter is the best timeout known to humankind. It captures our lightness and wisdom about what may be inexpressible. Laughter gives us a reset, relieving discomfort, suffering, and weariness by giving them air. It connects us deeply with others who share our knowledge of the truth—laughing together lightens our load.

Laughter has many health benefits. Dr. Norman Cousins cured his autoimmune disorder with daily doses of laughter. Laughter reduces stress hormones levels and inflammation. It makes us feel happier. It opens up our chests and makes us breathe more deeply. It literally vibrates the space of our fourth emotional center (see chapter nine—FLOW), moving grief and activating love. Laughter emboldens us through its spasmodic shock waves of understanding and wisdom. It helps us not take ourselves too seriously. All of our work is important, but we're all works in progress, and we're hilarious!

Art

Art is puttering, play, and creation in total present-moment engagement. Art is flow. Art is anything we set aside time and space to create for our pure enjoyment—painting, cooking, gardening, party planning, organizing . . . it's all art. It all pulls us out of ordinary time, engages our present-moment awareness, and provides necessary pause.

Meditation

We've talked about the benefits of meditation, but it's important to note here as well. Meditation is any form of quiet—still or active—contemplative activity that cultivates present-time awareness. Release of the past (regret, grief, rumination on tenacious stories) and the future (worry, fear) by its very nature soothes the nervous system, reduces stress, and calms the mind. Present-time awareness helps us become the compassionate observer, letting go of judgment for what we think and how we feel. It teaches us to find the space between our thoughts—space where possibilities arise.

Permission Slip: Permission to Rest, Pause, and Play

This is the first of several permission slips you'll write to yourself within this book, and I hope the first of many in your life! Permission slips call our power back. They're a tool we create ourselves to invite us to be our whole true selves and reclaim terrain—experiences, emotions, behaviors—that we need. They help us bypass the rules, judgments, and dictums of others. We know who we are. We know what we need. We give ourselves permission.

Write this on a piece of paper:

Dear [your name here],

Welcome home, dear one. Welcome home to rest, respite, pause, and play. Welcome to your body. Your breath. Your true nature.

I give you my full permission to rest. To release the past and present. To set aside time. To set aside all rules and competition. To be yourself. To do what you love. Or to do nothing at all. To just breathe and let go. To rest. You have my permission to just rest—to be. You deserve this.

Love, Me

LAST THOUGHTS

We've slept. We've learned to rest. We've found the audacity to give ourselves permission to pause.

But first we had to call our power back, didn't we? We had to let go and create time to claim our true priorities. We had to let love in, and find, nourish, and protect our strong centers.

Yah, we're badasses! We're beautiful, courageous beings creating our healing lives.

With all this, we've built the foundation for movement—and all the ways we inhabit our bodies well. Join me for our next domain: MOVE—Move, Balance, and Carry Yourself Well.

Chapter Six

MOVE

Move, Balance, and Carry Yourself Well

We've created space for our healing, courageously put ourselves first, and found our center. We've rested and restored. Life gifts us with so much, but now there's work to be done.

Our bodies—our greatest tools and teachers—must now carry us and those we love. We need our bodies strong, stable, nimble, and ready to engage. We must be in our bodies. For this we've got to show up for them through how we move, balance, and carry ourselves well.

WE'RE BORN TO MOVE

Movement is our legacy. It's really the whole reason for having a body at all—to move from one place to the next, to act on our intentions, to connect with one another. In so many ways, movement has allowed for our survival: to forage for food, hunt, move from place to place, and raise children. We've moved for play, love, and living in community among our tribes. As conscious, soulful beings, movement gets us closer to what inspires us and makes our lives richer. It allows us to interact with one another and exchange not just needed resources, but ideas, aspirations, and creative genius.

All body functions are shaped by how we move and hold ourselves in space. Movement, posture, and gravity result in definable "loads"—forces that act upon us physically—to which our bodies respond and adapt. The forces loading us through gravity, posture, and motion are delivered from point of contact all the way through to our cells where they are translated directly to our genes, creating adaptive shifts in how our genes are expressed. Genetic expression, therefore, responds to every aspect of how we move in space through loading. The effects of these shifts in our genetic expression (we refer to how the environment influences genetic expression as "epigenetics"), determine our size, shape, function, and state of health. Thus, the epigenetic effects of how we carry ourselves become a foundational point of personal control over our health and wellbeing.

We Are Designed for Optimal Loading through Movement and Posture

What constitutes the right amount of movement and exercise that leads to optimal loading of our cells and tissues? No one really knows for sure. But we can make reasonable approximations by looking at the behavior of our hunter-gatherer ancestors, whose genes are our legacy. They moved throughout their days out of necessity. They walked, ran, stood, sat, and squatted in different ways under a wide variety of loads all day long. They walked on nonuniform surfaces of varying grades, barefoot or on minimally covered feet (no pads or arch supports), slept on the ground, and worked for everything they needed— foraging, hunting, food preparation, fire tending, shelter, clothing, and tool creation, moving their homes from place to place, and carrying their children.

The children themselves began their physical training from day one, first by being carried on their parents' torsos, allowing them to develop strong, stable core musculature at an early age. They were further loaded by breast feeding, sleeping with their parents, and participating in foraging and activities of daily living as soon as they were mobile— much earlier than modern children. Even during sleep, without the mattresses and pillows we know today, their bodies adapted to greater challenges than we know.

Our remote ancestors' bodies adapted to the challenges of self-sufficiency and nomadic lifestyles. That adaptation included physiological processes required to support extensive movement and loading—energy production, detoxification, digestion and absorption of nutrients from food, circulation of blood and lymphatic fluids, brain and

HEAL KARYN SHANKS MD

neurological function, immune function, and the growth and strength of structural muscles, bones, and connective tissue. The higher loads our ancestors experienced favored heavy protection against oxidative stress—the potentially damaging price we pay for using oxygen to make energy—perhaps putting the brakes on much of the age-related deterioration we experience today.[17] The brain power required to manage the challenges of life—to problem solve, think creatively and quickly in the face of survival challenges— also benefitted from large loads, as virtually every aspects of brain function (size, number of connections between cells, learning, memory, and intelligence) is enhanced through optimal movement and loading.

The movement and loading of our ancestors are what "trained" our genetics and set the bar for what could be our optimal physiological functioning today. But while our DNA has not changed appreciably since our ancestors inhabited the earth, our environments and lifestyles have. As we all know, it's a dangerous mismatch.

Twenty-First Century Comfort and Convenience Take Their Toll

By contrast to our ancient ancestors, most of us in the twenty-first century sit at work, sit when we relax, sleep in our comfy beds, wear padded shoes with arch support, and maybe, just maybe, take an hour to exercise three to four times per week. We sit with our heads down and shoulders collapsed, focused on our laptops and small electronic devices. We move less in order to make room for our busy lives. When we do move, it's the same thing in the same way, repeated over and over again. We drive instead of walk or bike. We use elevators, escalators, automatic doors, and walk on carefully flattened and smoothed surfaces. We purchase prepackaged processed food instead of growing and preparing it at every step. We outsource most of our subsistence tasks to others and indulge in modern conveniences. On the whole, we move far less than we were designed to. And

---

[17] While many of our ancestors' life expectancy was cut short by higher infant mortality and deaths related to catastrophic injuries and illness (from which we are protected by modern medicine), there is archeological and anthropological evidence from hunter-gatherer populations that they were far healthier than we are.

because we're immobile for such long periods of time, we get weak and imbalanced, so when we do move, we move poorly and suffer the inevitable injuries, aches, and pains.

Virtually everything that ails us today—fatigue, pain, and chronic disease—can be traced back to how we move. Especially terrifying is the loss of cognitive function and mind potential that affects us in our daily lives—lost creativity, problem-solving ability, focus and follow through, and increased boredom—as well as abject deterioration of brain function. The epidemic of dementia and Alzheimer's is profoundly influenced by our culture's sedentary lifestyle.

It's not difficult to see why scientific studies of modern people have agreed that a sedentary lifestyle is dangerous to our health. Prolonged sitting is associated with increases in all causes of mortality, including cardiovascular disease, cancer, and diabetes, regardless of one's exercise program. While the benefits of regular exercise have also been proven, if the background activity of our daily lives is sedentary, that's bad. We were designed to be active and mobile through a range of positions all day.

Movement is also important for mental wellness. Exercise has been shown to have similar effectiveness as antidepressant medication for the treatment of depression and prevents relapse of depression after successful treatment. Exercise reduces anxiety, panic attacks, and irritability. It improves wellbeing, optimism, focus, concentration, and memory. It does so through its favorable effects on our brains, hormones, energy production, circulation, and detoxification.

I don't mean to scare you. All that bad news associated with a sedentary lifestyle points to some good news as well: movement is our untapped potential and opportunity for healing. We can eat well, sleep well, and avoid toxins, but without loading our bodies through a lifestyle of abundant and varied movement, our efforts will not reach the health and energy potential we seek.

THE DANGERS OF DECREASED MOBILITY AND REPETITIVE ACTION

As we've established, movement creates the loading that determines what we become: our shape, size, density, structure, composition, and physiological function. This complete package of the physical expression of our bodies results from the total of all loading incurred on our cells through movement and posture of our entire lives.

Wow. *The outcome of movement is us.*

How Movement Drives Physiology: Delivery of Oxygen to Cells

Let's drill down further into how movement shapes one of the foundational functions of the body: circulation of blood for carrying oxygen and nutrients to all body cells to support energy production and work.

Here's how it goes: The heart pumps blood, rich in oxygen just picked up from the lungs and nutrients from the gut, into the major blood vessels of the body. That blood moves forward as a result of force created by the heart's pumping and the pressure within the vessels, from large to successively smaller, as the blood gets closer to the tissues where the oxygen and nutrients are bound.

However, once the blood reaches the cells where it's needed, a different movement is required. That's right: the heart does not pump blood all the way to the cells. Our moving, contracting muscles do that! When muscles contract as we move, the very smallest blood vessel tributaries leading to the cells (called arterioles) open up, and subsequently release their contents into the capillary beds immediately surrounding the cells. This allows oxygen and nutrients to diffuse out of circulation and enter the cells, while waste products move out of the cells. The oxygen and nutrients are then used to create energy and support the work of the cells.

This is Why the Palace Guards Faint

There is no other way for this to happen. What happens when we stay in one place for long periods of time? Circulation is impaired. Oxygenation of the tissues is decreased. Energy production grinds to a halt in the immobile parts of the body. Cellular work and function decrease. Cellular death may ensue. It's a downstream process of negative consequences. A classic example of this is when the Queen of England's palace guards faint while standing ramrod straight at the castle gate for hours at a time. They don't faint from the heat or weakness, but from loss of blood flow and oxygenation to their brains and vital organs—the direct result of not moving. Fainting keeps them alive. To prevent fainting, they are actually taught to maintain blood flow through systematic contraction of their large muscle groups while not visibly moving.

Prolonged Fixed Postures Are Bad

Of course, those palace guards wouldn't necessarily be better off if they sat all day either. Consider the typical sitting posture—you might be sitting right now and can follow along with this closely.

Here's What Sitting Usually Looks Like Relative to Standing:

Your front body folds forward with ninety-degree angles at the hips and knees; your back body is proportionately lengthened with hamstrings (large muscles on the back of the thighs) flattened on the seat while legs below the knees drop vertically to the floor. Quadriceps (large muscles on the front of the thighs) and hip flexors (muscles that connect the upper leg to the torso to flex the hips) are shortened. Feet rest statically on the ground with ankles fixed in a static angle. Your back may be straight and supported by the chair, or tilted forward over a desk or table, perhaps leaning on outstretched arms at the elbows.

Both postures support the torso, releasing core engagement. Arms are likely supported, releasing engagement of the upper arms, shoulders, and upper back. With shoulders forward of the vertical (leaning over the desk, for instance), chest and back tuck back, chin and head protrude forward. Some people literally collapse the front of their bodies over the desks, laps, or workspaces especially when they are looking at a book or electronic device they are looking at. Focused engagement with the task in front of you likely leads to head and neck tilting forward (increasing the weight of the head relative to the neck) and jaw protruding.

What might this forwardly-closed, relatively fixed posture I've just described lead to over the course of many hours?

Three Problems Created by Prolonged Sitting (and All Prolonged Fixed Postures):

- inactivity (decreased loading),

- repetition of a static shape (loss of variation, which leads to selective decreased loading and adaptation), and

- loss of postural engagement and strength (loss of core strength).

Inactivity leads to global decline in energy production and expenditure, and generalized loss of strength. Lack of movement leads to decreased circulation and neurological input, particularly in those parts of the body compressed in a passive position—like the hamstrings.

Repetition of a static shape leads to problems resulting from adaptation to the position. In the case of prolonged sitting, the body gets used to the persistent practice of the sitting shape and adapts to make it easier and require less energy. The body works to maintain aspects of the practiced shape even when it attempts to transition into another shape, say from sitting to standing.

The release of core muscles associated with prolonged sitting leads to loss of postural engagement and the strength necessary to support alignment of the spine in an upright posture.

In addition, the persistently fixed muscles are excessively shortened or lengthened in their practiced positions: the chest and abdominal muscles, arms, hip flexors, and quadriceps in the front body are excessively shortened; while the neck, back, and hamstrings continue to be excessively lengthened. This front to back configuration tends to persist even as one transitions to standing up and walking. That's why people who sit all day hunched over a desk as part of their occupation, tend to move in a partially sitting shape when they get up to walk. Take a close look at people as they walk down the street: they're tilted forward with forwardly flexed heads, shoulders, hips, and knees, falling forward with each step.

When Balance and Efficiency Work Against Us

This is the balance and equilibrium imperative of nature—if you spend the majority of your waking hours sitting, that's what the body will remodel itself to do as efficiently as possible—keeping you in that shape with as little energy expenditure as possible. Then anything else you choose to do—standing, walking, running, working out at the gym—will be limited by what your body redesigned itself for.

I want to reemphasize that *any* prolonged position can be damaging. If prolonged sitting is the new smoking,[18] as talked about recently in the press, then prolonged standing is just as bad. It's great to find ways to accomplish what we normally sit to do by standing. For instance, standing desks are a good idea. But, if you're like me, when I get focused on a writing project, I forget to move whether I'm sitting or standing, which doesn't offer any more benefit than sitting the whole time. The point here is that any prolonged posture immobilizes us and leads to adaptation and loss of strength. We're meant to move, to shift how we're loading our bodies, not to become fixed in one place.

Prolonged Postures Increase Our Vulnerability to Injury and Dysfunction

So, we know that immobility is bad for a lot of reasons. But let's look more closely to really understand why this is true.

The adaptation to sitting we've discussed—or any other fixed position—results in the muscles becoming weak and losing their ability to create force. The joints around which the muscles work lose range of motion because of imbalanced muscle length and strength. If we then ask our muscles to go to work—say by going to the gym after being at the office all day, or going home to play vigorously with our kids—we do so with less stability at our joints and less capacity to safely move them through their full range. We may end up excessively loading the weakened, destabilized, and restricted joint, while recruiting adjacent joints (that may not be built for the load) to assist us—they help us cheat our limitations to reach our desired end range. This scenario leads to strains, tears, and a world of hurt.

In addition to loss of strength and mobility, the forwardly closed position of sitting (or limited position of any persistently fixed and immobile position) constricts the circulation of blood, lymph, and tissue fluid through those structures, limiting oxygen

─────────────────────────────

[18] Recent research has shown that prolonged sitting is as harmful to health as smoking. See references in the further resources section at the end of this book.

and nutrient delivery, and impairing energy production. We've already talked about the dangers of stagnation of blood flow, but the same concept applies to lymphatic flow and tissue fluid. This stagnation of fluids resulting from lack of movement leads to less fuel arriving to the cells for energy production, as well as buildup of toxins and irritants that we fail to clear out.

Adding to all this, a muscularly contracted torso limits full excursion of the diaphragm and chest wall, diminishing breath capacity and oxygen availability. This combination—decreased circulation and oxygen supply—adds to deficiency of function in the face of the need for energy and detoxification.

And it keeps going! The shallow breathing associated with prolonged sitting leads to loss of diaphragmatic contraction, which stimulates the vagus nerve—a powerful neurological mediator of the parasympathetic nervous system (PNS). This has all the implications for energy, mood, and resilience to stress that we discussed in chapter five.

Finally, prolonged sitting tethers us to a posture that is defensive and guarded. As we'll discuss more in a bit, our postures affect presence—how we emotionally and psychologically inhabit our bodies. As we'll see, sustained forwardly folded postures measurably decrease courage, confidence, and ability to engage in a positive way with others. The loss of muscle control, balance, and stability of prolonged sitting adds up to feeling and behaving less empowered.

PRESENCE—EMPOWERMENT THROUGH EMBODIED MOVEMENT

We *live* in our bodies. They're not just the repositories of our biology, they're *us*—minds, emotions, and spirits. But we can zip our awareness out of our bodies. We can move through our lives, taking action and creating postures that are not conscious. We can live without paying attention, disconnected from our thoughts and feelings, and lose connection to the guidance of our strong center within. When we are not present, when we lose our embodied presence, we lose control of our greatest potential strength.

Presence is how we inhabit our bodies and use them to engage with present time. We do this through attention to movement, posture, and sensations. At the core of presence is the strong, nimble, conscious movement we've talked about that extends from the strong, resilient center we created in chapter four. Presence that is mindful, purposeful, reverent, and embodied is powerful. It makes us electric with connection as it anchors us to present-moment awareness, attuning us to our true selves and real lives.

Embodied presence helps us feel more confident. It strengthens and calms. It elevates our capacity to engage with others. It allows us to perform—our work, our play, and our daily chores—with greater depth and aptitude. Consciously inhabiting our bodies—when we move, when we sit, when we play—is not just good for our bodies, it allows greater richness of the human experience.

My Story

I started running as a teenager, inspired by the notion that I could replace bad habits with something more positive and possibly good for me. It was awful at first, and I hated it, but I stubbornly stuck with it—I desperately wanted to feel better. I started with one block, the next day two, gradually, painstakingly increasing my distance. It was not fun as I ached and gasped for breath, but I was intrigued as I experienced the faintest ripple of empowerment when I accomplished the grueling task set before me each day.

Before I knew it, I was running miles rather than blocks. My energy was up. My confidence soared. I felt really, really good about myself. Some of this was a sense of accomplishment for succeeding at something really hard that I'd never imagined myself doing. But I also felt different about my body in a new and strange way. It was like I was *in* my body for the first time. I felt like I *existed*. I could feel myself through my effort and work and soreness. And, unexpectedly, I felt more whole, and more present to myself, my life, and the world around me.

Running was a revelation. It literally saved me at a very difficult time in my life. It reduced my anxiety, cleared my mind, and helped me focus and concentrate on my schoolwork. It gave me a sense of accomplishment and worth. It became my first true love as it connected me deeply to nature and my environment while I pounded the streets and trails of my favorite running paths. Running kept me entertained, but also grounded, more stable, less stressed, and more courageous.

Since all I did was run (and run and run) for many years, I accumulated injuries. It led to excessive stress on my body from repetitive geometry and forces: Remember our lesson about vulnerability to injury from prolonged fixed postures? The same is true for prolonged, limited, repetitive movement. I learned the virtues and necessity of variety. I've since tried many types of exercise and movement. I found that I hated the repetition of exercise classes that went through the same routine every time. And the machines and gym regimens were tedious and boring. I needed nature, purpose, and diversity!

These days I do lots of things to stay active. I try to move more in my daily life and reduce sitting. I transitioned to a standing desk, though, as we've discussed, I tend to stay just as fixed as I would be sitting—I'm working on that. I also go to the gym where I work on strength, power, mobility, and balance. The movements are purposeful—they are about function, strength, and meaningful performance rather than just lifting weights up and down in a boring repetitive fashion. I work on the structure of a new movement, using the body in its intended positions, progress it, and gradually develop the skill and strength.

I also do yoga and hike in the woods (yes, on uneven trails, going both up and down hills). These hikes are more inward leaning, restorative, and body opening, but all of my activities take me on an inward journey, just in different ways. Each one is a meditative discipline calling me to greater presence and attention to myself and what's around me. I love being strong and stable in my body, mastering a skill that takes me beyond what I thought was possible. The pull-ups, toes to bar, and Ardha Chandrasana (half-moon pose) all take me there, and I carry this into my everyday life. The deep embodiment practice makes me feel more alive, clearer, and open to the possibilities of the day, expecting the best. I am more vital and vibrant because of my daily discipline of movement practices, and for me this is their greatest value. The health benefits are wonderful, especially as I age, but it's their nourishing effects on my wellbeing that sustains my hard work and discipline to do them.

Using Movement for Personal Empowerment

Just like I learned as a teenager, simple, regular movement can make you feel like the better version of yourself, more connected to everything, more present, and empowered.

Yoga

Yogis have known for centuries that specific kinds of movement increase awareness, strengthen mindful presence, and open us to a deeper level of wisdom and experience. Yoga instructors teach that by moving our bodies and holding postures, we not only stretch and strengthen our bodies, but just as important, we transform our minds and emotions. Some poses help us feel more open hearted and courageous. Others help us feel strong and centered. Still others open us to gratitude or help us surrender and let go. Holding yoga poses and using breath, keeps us more aware of our bodies, tethering us to the present moment. We can accomplish this very same experience of present moment awareness through many other forms of movement when done mindfully, like gardening, walking in the woods, working out at the gym, or mowing the lawn.

Power Poses

There is science to support the idea that it's all one big feedback loop—our minds tell our bodies to do something and the action of doing that thing changes how our minds experience them. This is true not just when doing yoga or exercising, but in all the movements of our daily lives. In her book, *Presence*, social scientist Amy Cuddy describes her elegant research about how we carry ourselves—how we move, stand, and speak— influences our sense of power and courage. She shows how positive postures make us *feel* more positive about ourselves, which influences our actions and willingness to take risks, to stand up for ourselves, and to present ourselves in a confident manner. These positive postures lead to physiological changes that support assertiveness (increased testosterone) and calm (lower cortisol).

If you've seen Dr. Cuddy's TED Talk, you will be familiar with the "high power poses" presented as simple ways to accomplish the open posture that lends itself to greater power and presence. These include what we call, the star fish pose in yoga—stand tall, heart open, arms up with hands at forty-five degrees, face tilted upward. Her research demonstrated that this and other power poses used for just a minute at a time, compared with more closed poses helped subjects feel more powerful, confident, and willing to take risks. Her conclusion: "The body shapes the mind."

Dangers of "iPosture"

Cuddy warns about the dangers of closed, defensive postures, one of which she refers to as "iPosture," or "iHunch," the hunched over, heart closed, shoulders collapsed posture of the twenty-first-century human being striving to improve productivity and efficiency through use of small electronic devices such as smart phones, tablet devices, and laptops. Her research reveals that even short stretches of this activity reduced assertiveness, perhaps counteracting efforts to improve our lives.

Mind-Body Presence Using Active Imagination

But here's something really mind blowing about this body-mind feedback loop: Cuddy extended her work to people who have disabilities and are unable to stand in an open power posture. She asked the subjects to *imagine* themselves in power poses and then describe how they felt. They used descriptors very similar to the standing subjects, such as "open, strong, grounded, confident, comfortable, and poised." Their experimental counterparts, who imagined themselves in the more contracted low-power poses, reported feeling "awkward, tense, scared, lonely, vulnerable, threatened, and uncomfortable."

Our minds, our bodies, and our spirits are all one. Not just in a metaphysical, hypothetical "new age" way. But in a real physical way that makes a lot of sense. If you think about how an organism as complex as ourselves has evolved to deal with the world, it's beautiful!

But it's also a challenge. As with so much you'll discover in this book, this process is always going on whether you realize it or not. The challenge is to use it, to direct it, to be active about it. Being passive about it doesn't mean it's not happening. It just means you have no control over any of the outcome. Taking control of your movement means you direct the course of your life—you step into the potential you choose.

Self-Reflection Exercise: Where Are You?

Close your eyes. Where are you located? You know, the you-you, the real you?

Are you in your head? Heart? Gut? Above or outside of your body somewhere?

Write your answer down. It will be very interesting to remember your response after you practice the exercises that follow.

When was the last time you listened to what your body had to tell you? What did it say? Hunger, pain, fatigue? Anger, irritability, happiness?

The following exercises will help you to become a deeper listener and observer of yourself. Your perspective will shift depending on where you are in your body.

Conscious Breathing Movement

Breathing is movement. It's the part of our movement that supports the energy we need to move and function in space. It moves blood and lymph, aids digestive movement, and calms the nervous system.

Breathing is a primary rhythm of the body that occurs continuously, as long as we are alive, without needing conscious input. But even though it can continue without thought or effort, this doesn't mean we are making the most of it. With conscious input, breath becomes a tool for mental and physical awareness and nervous system recovery.

Conscious breathing both calms and energizes. It focuses, sustains intensity, and moves emotional energy. Focusing on breathing can guide us out of the past and the stories that tether us there. It helps us be in our present-moment experience, while supporting us through the intensity of it.

Deep breathing grounds us into our bodies, providing respite from the dominance of overly analytical minds, connecting us more deeply to our more primal intuitive intelligence. This movement out of our heads and more into our bodies makes us feel more balanced and whole. It relieves anxiety and enhances our sense of connection to ourselves. And as we've seen, it lends itself to confidence and courage.

Physically, breath extracts oxygen from the air and moves it to the blood, from where it is transported to our cells and converted to energy. Exhalation blows off carbon dioxide, the end product of cellular energy production. Diaphragmatic breathing—conscious, slow, deep—stimulates the vagus nerve, leading to parasympathetic nervous system stimulation to calm and slow us down. It helps sustain us through intensity and difficulty and supports neutral, present-moment observation of our sensations and emotions.

Breath integrates all of us—body, mind, and spirit. When we learn to breathe deeply *into* our bodies, we become more aware of ourselves as *inhabiting* our bodies. We become more aware of the sensations and emotions that reside there, observing their location, flow, or where they get stuck. In this way breath delivers the wisdom of our bodies right into our present-time consciousness.

The following is an exercise for embodied breathing to help you become anchored within your body using a simple breath and awareness techniques. It's a long one but well worth the practice and will become fast and second nature as you use it.

Exercise: Embodied Breathing

Most of us spend so much time in our heads, it can be challenging to even find our bodies.

This elegant and simple exercise pulls our attention into our bodies so we become more connected to present-moment sensations and feelings. It's a practice that is wonderful for grounding—the full experience of inhabiting and "living" inside the body. It is a calming and revitalizing practice that I love to use at the beginning of a meditation practice or any time I need to come in from the clouds.

There are many versions of embodied breathing practices, often called "body scans." I particularly like a version by Judith Blackstone, who teaches inhabiting the body as a way to "attune" to our fundamental "essential self" consciousness. Through the practice of inhabiting the body with our attention, she teaches that we learn to live within the body automatically, without having to work at it. In time it becomes an effortless transformation of the way we experience ourselves and our environment. My exercise is inspired by the many versions of body scans I've practiced over the years

The description for this exercise is long—to walk you through the details of mindful embodiment practice. But once you go through it a time or two it will be a snap, perhaps taking you just seconds or a few minutes to accomplish.

This exercise can be done sitting, standing, or lying down. Close your eyes or softly focus your gaze on the ground in front of you. If sitting, be on your sit bones on a chair or cushion, spine straight, shoulders over hips, chin slightly tucked. If lying down, tuck your shoulder blades underneath you and turn your palms upward. Make sure you are warm enough and comfortable.

If sitting, bring your thumb, pointer, and middle fingers together and let your hands rest in your lap. This hand positioning allows for deeper excursion of the diaphragm, which facilitates the deepest breathing. If standing, let your hands fall gently to your sides and create the same hand position as for sitting. You may also bring your palms lightly together in front of the heart center to activate sensation in the palms. Make sure your shoulders are back and heart is open.

Take a few deep breaths and let it all go. Just be. Relax. Be present in your body.

Now breathe into the tips of your toes. Breathe in there and let the breath just settle in the tips of the toes. Let the in-breath draw your awareness and energy into your toes. When you breathe out, concentrate your breath there. Be in your toes. Continue to breathe in and out of the tips of your toes until you feel you are there. If you'd like, send a positive message to your toes. Express your gratitude for how they help stabilize you or how they wiggle so well. The physiology of gratitude and positive affirmations will deliver nourishing blood flow and reduce negative inputs to your body.

Next, breathe in through the tips of your toes and now extend the breath up to the balls of your feet. Again, be there. Breathe in awareness and energy to the balls of your feet. Breathe out to concentrate the breath and energy there. You are fully aware and present in the tips of your toes to the balls of your feet. Be aware of both sides of your body. Be content to work on this until it feels comfortable and you are there, in the tips of your toes and the balls of your feet on both sides.

Next, breathe in through the tips of your toes, extending to the balls of your feet, continuing up to the ankles of both feet. Breathe in. Lead your awareness and energy to the ankles. Breathe out. Concentrate it there. Be in your toes, feet, and ankles.

Now continue this practice, ascending from the tips of your toes all the way to your hips. Take as much time as you need to fully feel yourself in your body.

Now move to the torso. Start with the floor of the pelvis. Move your breath up the legs and concentrate it in the pelvic floor. Move your breath, awareness and energy into your pelvic floor. Be there. Expand your breath and energy there. Gradually move to the pelvic bowl that includes your hips and sacrum. Then move to your torso and solar plexus, expanding and concentrating your breath there, then to the heart center, and eventually to your head. Fill your pelvic floor, pelvic bowl, torso, solar plexus, heart center, and center of your head with your breath, awareness, and energy. Let yourself settle there. Be in your limbs and head and torso simultaneously. Let your energy contract and expand with your breath. Feel your awareness and your whole self in your body.

Now use your breath to bring your awareness into your arms, starting with the fingertips and gradually moving up into the shoulders. Try to simultaneously move your breath from the toes on up. This may be a challenge and will take some practice. Don't try too hard. Work on awareness of your entire body at the same time. Be there.

Continue to breathe awareness and energy in from the tips of your toes and fingers, permeating your whole body. In-breath pulls energy in. Out-breath concentrates energy, plumping up your body with energy and awareness. Be in your body. Be fully in your body. Continue this practice until you feel the presence of yourself deeply within your body.

Congratulations! This is a very challenging practice in the beginning. In time and with practice, you will be able to accomplish this entire exercise in just a few minutes. You *may also be able to put yourself in your body instantaneously, with simple intention and a single breath or two. You can use it as a prelude to a longer meditation or do it in an instant as a timeout during a busy day. It is a great way to recharge and reconnect to yourself so you can move through your day and your life from a more self-aware, grounded, and stable position.*

Embodiment Science—Flow

Embodiment makes our minds work better. We solve those unsolvable problems. Conjure those brilliant ideas. And we perform most anything we've practiced at our best. How does that work? Beyond present-moment awareness, how does conscious engagement of our bodies help us think and function better in our bodies?

Flow.

Flow is a term popularized within the arena of elite athletics to describe the state of optimal body-mind-environment alignment that leads to peak performance. Flow is available to us all. People in a flow state consciously inhabits their bodies while disengaging just enough from their thoughts (and the judgments and stories that can get in the way) to perform at a higher level.

In his book *The Rise of Superman*, Steven Kotler speaks of "deep embodiment" as a necessary ingredient to flow. He teaches that a key part of how we get out of our heads (and away from the distraction of stories) to achieve flow is to overwhelm the brain with enough sensory input from the body to quiet the excessive thinking that gets in the way.

The Power of Hypofrontality

Deep embodiment capitalizes on the enormous amount of sensory information coming into the brain from the body and the environment all around. Over fifty percent of all sensory input to the brain comes from the hands, feet, and face. Another large percentage is generated from neurons involved in balance, movement, and proprioception (our sense of where we are in space). When engaging the full body, the tsunami of sensory input to the brain overwhelms its ability to process it all, leading to the state Kotler refers to as "hypofrontality," a state in which we overwhelm the analytical, logical prefrontal cortex with so much sensory data that we remove its control and interference with the complex activities we want to excel at. It's like a self-induced temporary pre-frontal lobotomy.

If this idea of intentionally shifting the focus of the brain seems a bit strange, realize we do this unintentionally all the time. Think about the last time you were deeply engrossed in a movie at your local theater. As the plot intensified and the heroes had to deal with it, I doubt you were in the slightest bit aware of the folks in the theater with you. Our brain shifts focus all the time. Hypofrontality, or flow, or being in the zone, are just different names for using specific tools to shift the focus of our brains. Of the tools available to us, deep embodiment is one of the most powerful.

In the very same way, we all can also use the strategy of deep embodiment through hypofrontality to also better access our wisdom—our mind flow. We do this by getting into our bodies through conscious, intentional movement.

Embodied Walking

Nothing shakes me lose like walking, especially in nature. Arms swinging, legs reaching out, climbing, breathing, letting go. It's always transformative. Worries and concerns dissipate with each step. Confusion and suffering—even the deep tenacious kind—shift into something less intense and more clear. Solutions rise up as I wander and meander. Problems are often miraculously solved. Articles and book chapters are written. Or maybe I just commune with the birds and trees and deer and feel amazed.

Walking has been called the "controlled art of falling." When we walk, we intentionally unbalance ourselves and start to fall forward. Then we catch ourselves and do it again. Each fall-catch is a step. Each step is part of a journey. So conscious walking is complex. While balancing our physical, controlled falling, our brains are also noticing sounds, the smells, the owl in the tree that we didn't see until we were upon it. With embodied walking, we disengage a bit with our overwrought analytical brain.

Exercise: Embodied Walking Practice

Dressed comfortably, with minimalist shoes (so your feet can spread out and really feel the ground beneath you—more on feet in a bit!), take off for a walk. Let your senses remain free. Avoid unnecessary distractions—put your phone away, listen only to the sounds of your environment. Walk where you feel safe and, if possible, where there is more of the natural world (trees, grasses, birds, and animals) and less of the human developed world (cars, cement, noise).

First, engage your core as you stride. Tune in to and turn on your legs, the large gluteal (buttock) muscles and abdominal muscles. Feel their strength. Walk with the strength of your core. Slow down. Breathe.

Once you've practiced walking with a turned-on core, begin to let go. Breathe deeply and let your arms swing naturally. Sink into the rhythm. Sense the dynamic equilibrium you create with your engaged core yet relaxed rhythm.

Feel your body. Feel your feet against the ground. Feel the contours of the ground beneath you. Listen. Hear the sounds of the trees, the birds, and the leaves crackling under your feet. Smell the dampness of the leaves and the flowers. See the colors of the grasses, the sparkle of the sunlight against the water, the clouds in the sky. Perhaps you can taste the sea salt or the cleanness of the air.

This is embodied walking—being in your body and present time awareness as you move. This creates flow. Flow brings peace even as you execute a very complex task. This peace through embodiment opens the doors to expanded awareness and creative thinking.

Embodiment Moves Emotions: Moving and Shaking

A mentor of mine in the field of mind-body medicine, Dr. James Gordon, works with people from around the world who have suffered deep trauma, teaching them mind-body skills to help them recover. He once spoke of working with a group of young girls from

Bosnia who had experienced unspeakable horror at the hands of Serb forces, who committed rape, torture, and murder as part of their ethnic cleansing campaign in the 1990s.

Dr. Gordon described how quiet and scared the young girls were, huddled together, bodies stiff, unable to communicate. He started their work together with a simple moving and shaking exercise. He put on music, had them all stand up together and begin by moving and shaking their bodies, starting with the feet and hands, jumping up and down, gradually getting their whole bodies involved. The sheer silliness of this exercise was infectious, and as the girls got moving, they started to giggle and look at one another. Their bodies began to release the tension they held, and the energy of their emotions began to flow with their movements. In just a few minutes they were present and engaged within the group.

Dr. Gordon had a group of us at one of his trainings do the same exercise. It was hilarious, got us all into our bodies, and set the tone of relaxed embodiment for the remainder of the session. Dr. Gordon's story is a profound example of the embodied nature of our emotions and how accessible they can be to physical approaches, especially when direct exploration may be too painful.[19]

BECOME A CONSCIOUS MOVER— GET HEALTHY AND FLOW

"The obstacle is the path."

—Zen proverb

Get Ready—Move More, Sit Less, Engage with Life

You don't have to become an athlete to benefit hugely from movement. You don't have to *exercise* at all. I'm not saying exercise is bad. In fact, it can be fantastic. But I want to make

---

[19] We'll be taking a deeper journey into the emotional realm in chapter nine, FLOW.

a clear distinction before we move on: *movement is not the same as exercise.*

Exercise is a subset of movement. It has value—we know that. It can be therapeutic, allowing us to work on strength and balance we've lost as a result of our sedentary lifestyles. Exercise can supplement daily activities and address injuries. And it can be fun. But it is never a substitute for the wide range of movements and behaviors that support us throughout our days.

The real challenge is not how to find time to go to the gym. The real challenge is to figure out how to move more in the course of our daily lives. This means how to give up sitting, how to stand more, how to create new and innovative opportunities to move and experience a multitude of loads and sensations.

We Start with Letting Go of Old Stories

To begin, we build on what we've already started in previous chapters and exercises: to move more and sit less, we have to let go of our old stories:

I can't.

I don't have time.

I'm not worthy (of attention to my own self-care).

And let's add a couple more that I hear all the time from my clients:

It's inconvenient.

It's uncomfortable.

What are these stories we tell ourselves really saying? We're spoiled! Our comfortable and convenience-driven lives have made us wimpy and soft. The ease we seek decreases the challenge, the loading, and the good stress we need to strengthen and remodel our bodies and fortify our center. We know this is a huge issue. And we've all learned the ramifications of living physically easy lives: it leads to a world of hurt. As we've discussed, most of what ails us has come about as a result of our behavior.

So, what can we do?

Then, Slow Down!

Slow down? Yes, we've talked about this before. So, we're all experts at slow by now, right? We all get the point, right? We have to go slow to observe, to feel, to *be*. And that's what conscious moving and embodiment are all about. No short cuts. No hacks.

Move into Your Feet

That's right, start with your feet. The feet you stand on the earth with. The feet that move you forward. The feet that keep you balanced. We need robust feet to stand tall and move strong. But our lifestyle of comfort and immobility has taken its toll on us. The shoes we wear with arch support, thick cushions, immobilizing structure, and even heels (yikes!), destabilize and make our feet (and us!) weak.

When I was growing up, we went barefoot constantly—outdoors all summer and indoors in the winter. We played in the yard, the woods, around the neighborhood. We jumped and skipped and skated and rode our bikes. I rarely wore shoes and seldom sat down (the days before electronics!). In my twenties I began wearing running shoes with extensive arch support and cushioning—that's when my problems began. Foot pain, plantar fasciitis, and knee pain. I blamed it on the running, yet when I switched to minimalist shoes for athletic endeavors, and got back to walking barefoot, those problems all resolved and have never returned.

Feet, just like the rest of the body, need to be engaged to stay strong. Our feet are highly complex with many bones, joints, muscles and connective tissue. When we wear "supportive" footwear, we significantly immobilize them. This leads to loss of strength, mass, and function that impairs their ability to carry us around and keep us stable. The stresses and strains that evolve as we wear shoes lead to injuries. After those injuries we tend to coddle our feet even more, which may feel better temporarily, but doesn't give us sustainable solutions to our problems by addressing the underlying causes.

Likewise, many of us wear shoes with heels, placing further stress on our feet. No matter how high they are—though higher ones are certainly worse—heels alter our bodies' alignment all the way up to the neck and head. Heels are terrible for our feet and exacerbate the full-body trauma created by our sitting lifestyle by forcing unnatural shapes. When our feet are not in close contact with the ground beneath us, (sorry, platform shoes don't solve the heel problem!), we lose the exquisite sensory information (like proprioception—how we neurologically know where we are in space) that keeps us steady and safe.

Working with your feet opens the doors to the embodiment, self-awareness, strength, and stability most of us seek. And it will resolve a multitude of problems that may surprise you through creation of a more robust platform from which to move.

If you suffer from foot pain, or are unused to spending much time barefoot, start this process slowly. Initially, spend just a few minutes at a time, standing and walking barefoot. Gradually work yourself up to spending most of your indoor, and perhaps some of your outdoor time, without shoes.

It took me many months to work up to freedom from wearing shoes—I'm at the point where I'm always barefoot inside my house. I also take my shoes off at work frequently and walk around my yard without shoes. I remain barefooted at the gym and wear minimalist athletic shoes for walks in the woods—no arch support or cushion, just a bit of rubber under the sole. Do I completely avoid heels? Mostly, but not completely. I love the look of them, though I hate anything over an inch or two. They're not only uncomfortable for my feet, hips, and back, but they make me feel ungrounded—I always feel desperate to kick them off to feel like myself again.

So, ditch your shoes and wake up your feet! Do it slowly and mindfully. When barefoot, put your awareness into your feet. Spread your toes and stretch them against the floor. Consciously allow your feet to hold and balance you from all aspects—toes, front, back, and sides. Briefly stand on your tippy toes, then your heels. See what that feels like. Use your feet to pick up a tissue, small towel, or ball. Generate sensation by rolling the bottoms of your feet out on a tennis or lacrosse ball, massaging them gently.

Stand Well

We must stand well to prepare us for strong, stable, balanced movement. Standing well is a skill which takes instruction and practice, especially for adults whose bodies have lost the feel of optimal stability, strength, and functional body mechanics due to lack of movement and excessive sitting with poor posture. It's not enough to simply stop sitting. When we attempt to stand after prolonged sitting, our standing posture tends to continue to reflect the shape of sitting. The various bends (knees, hips, pelvis, shoulders, neck and head) persist, destabilizing the intended standing postures.

What should standing well look like? Start by standing in front of a full-length mirror so you can see your front and sides. Stand with feet pointed directly forward, hip-distance apart. Stand up straight. Drop your arms to your sides, palms facing forward. Tuck your chin slightly and lift your heart up and out. Now, stick your butt out behind you. Then, squeeze your gluteal muscles (your butt) and tuck your pelvis underneath you without thrusting your legs forward. Feel the strength of your butt, legs, and abs. We want pelvis and spine in good alignment. Do all this while still maintaining heart out and shoulders back.

Now, feel your feet against the ground beneath you, strengthen your legs, engage your thighs, and lengthen the sides of your torso. Inflate your midback with each breath without changing your spinal alignment.

These cues place you into a variation of a standing pose in yoga, called Tadasana, or mountain pose. Deceptively, it's one of the hardest poses in yoga because it asks us to stand correctly when our bodies are accustomed to sitting, followed by standing poorly in a partially sitting posture. This simple practice takes us out of our comfort zone. However, with enough practice it will reestablish the alignment and balance we are meant to have while standing on our two feet.

Standing well is the base from which to move to other life "poses." Standing is not naturally a static position. We were no more meant to stand all day than we were to sit. Standing initiates movement. From this basic standing form, we can shift from one leg to the other, take off into a walk, adjust our leg position, move from standing to sitting or squatting, and prepare for more complex and strenuous movements. Standing is home base. We always come back to it.

Sit Well

"No chairs make for short meetings."

—Henry Ford

Sitting is our modern adaptation to a more comfortable lifestyle and more sedentary work. While prolonged sitting is one the most lethal of all our behaviors, it's so entrenched in our culture that we can't always avoid it. There are times we must sit.

So, we can learn to sit well. There is much we can do to optimize the sitting posture. As a physician-consultant, I must sit with my patients. This is the most comfortable, relaxed, and safe posture for the lengthy conversations we engage in. It is never ideal but I have found ways to mitigate some of the problems that can arise for both my clients and me, such as stiffness and fatigue.

First of all, I sit well: on a comfortable seat, squarely on my sit bones, back straight, arms comfortably at my sides, chin slightly tucked. I have a tendency to stick my chin and head forward while listening intently, which can lead to pain at the base of my neck later on. I try very hard to keep my neck in good alignment. If I forget, my sore neck will let me know!

Like all other postures, sitting well is not meant to be static. We need to vary the shape of our sitting posture. I like to fidget. I cross and uncross my legs, sit with legs even and straight ahead, move the placement of my seat around, move my arms around, shift my pelvis and head around. Of course, these movements are happening subtly and somewhat unconsciously. With practice and self-awareness I have become attuned to my alignment and need for movement and I make adjustments frequently, trying not to provide comic relief for my clients. I also create times within lengthier consultations for us to open up our posture by standing up, taking a bathroom break, and moving around. I like to take a quick star fish pose with arms up overhead and head back. We then get up to move to another room for the physical exam and reconvene back to our seats when finished. Once my client has left, I take my shoes off and remain standing. I go to my next tasks and purposefully remain standing to counterbalance the effects of so much sitting.

The overarching goal with sitting is to not stay absolutely static, allowing for as many variations in the forces acting upon us as possible.

HEAL KARYN SHANKS MD

Outside of my consultation room, I can vary my sitting posture even more. I've recently begun to sit on the floor more, changing up my position frequently. This was really hard in the beginning because my body was no longer accustomed to the hard floor or my haunches! Initially I felt stiff and sore and could only tolerate positions for a short period of time. But like anything, with practice, I'm gradually becoming more nimble.

Practice Restorative Postures to Unwind Prolonged Sitting

For those times when there is simply no choice but to sit for extended periods, here are three simple restorative postures that can be done for just minutes each day to help unwind the persistent forwardly folded posture caused by sitting. These are safe to do by almost everyone.

Corpse Pose

The full expression of corpse pose, also known as Shavasana in the yoga tradition, is to be lying flat on your back, against the ground, without props, arms out and bent at the elbows ("cactus arms") or by your side with hands facing upward. Using just the force of gravity, this pose gently opens the hips and shoulders while allowing the knees, hip flexors, and lower back to gradually drop into a more elongated resting position. Initially you may need a pillow under your head or bolster under your knees to prevent discomfort. Work gradually to reduce the size of your props, eventually eliminating them altogether.

Cobra Pose

The full expression of this pose is front lying on your stomach, legs stretched out behind you, with palms flat against the ground in front of you, arms straight, heart open, head facing forward or upward. Cobra pose is more intense that corpse pose, with more emphasis on opening of the hips, hip flexors, and chest—the exact opposite of what happens with sitting. This pose may be modified early on by resting on elbows, with forearms extending forward on the ground in front of them, palms against the ground (sphinx pose). Or you may start with a simple front lying position with forehead resting on stacked hands, working toward a very small, gentle rising of the chest from the ground, gradually working toward the full pose.

Child's Pose

The full expression of this pose is what we see in babies and small children: front lying on folded legs, knees facing forward, torso sinking in between them, with arms stretched forward and forehead on the ground or resting on stacked hands, or arms resting along the sides. The torso and hips relax on the folded haunches.

While at first glance this pose seems to fold forward, like sitting, it actually allows gravity and the weight of your body to gently stretch the tops of your feet and fronts of the legs—the shins and large muscles of the thighs—which are all shortened by sitting. It also passively allows for opening of the chest and shoulders. Forehead may rest on the ground or on a pillow formed by the hands. Forehead may also rest on the ground with arms resting at sides or stretched out in front for greater shoulder opening.

Balance Well

In chapter four, we talked about inner balance coming from our strong center. That paradigm of balance is part and parcel of physical balance. In addition to moving more, varying our movements, and learning to align our bodies well as we sit, stand, and walk it's also good to work on movements that challenge our stability. Feeling unstable begets emotions of vulnerability and not feeling safe in our own bodies—and we *are* less safe, at increased risk for falls, injuries, and bone fractures.

Try this: balance on one leg in a static position. Can you do it without holding on to something to steady yourself? If not, that's your starting place. Stand next to a chair or wall. Lift up your leg and balance on the other. Hold the position for thirty seconds and gradually increase over time. Work toward balancing on one leg without holding on for support. Do both sides. Gradually increase your time. As you become proficient, try standing on something squishy, like a pillow or pad. Make it harder. Can you balance while looking up at the ceiling? Can you close your eyes?

What else challenges your balance? Some may feel greatly challenged by moving from walking on a flat sidewalk to a bumpy trail in the woods. Or squatting down to your haunches and getting back up without support. Or sitting on the floor, then rising to standing without using your hands as leverage to assist you. Being able to get up from a seated position on the ground to full standing without using support has actually been shown to correlate with overall health, functional status, and mortality.

Whatever that challenge is for you, walk into it. Embrace it. Your brain will love it. With practice, your balance—and power—will soar.

Looking for a great way to work on strength, alignment, balance, breath, and embodiment all in one practice? Try yoga. Yoga combines mindfully executed postures in a way that allows us to work on all aspects of conscious movement.

Moderate Exercise and High Intensity Interval Training (HIIT)

While exercise cannot be a substitute for daily movement, it can be an important part of our lives—it can be fun, therapeutic, and social. I'm a huge fan! Moderate exercise (like walking thirty to sixty minutes) performed every day, and HIIT, frequent but short bursts of high intensity activity, several times weekly for just a few minutes has been shown to increase protection from oxidative stress, improve energy production, reduce inflammation, and increase all measures of strength, stability, and performance. Not only do these activities make us healthier, they improve mood and psychology through favorable effects on hormones and neurochemistry and contribute to the power of embodiment.

How to Address Challenges

As you practice and develop your movements, they will all become easier. Your body will adapt to the new balance and you will find more flow with your movements. But no path worth walking is entirely smooth. There will be challenges. Here's how to address the big ones.

Change It Up

In the course of our daily lives, it is ideal to use our whole body, varying our activities to challenge and mobilize us in different ways. The idea is not to do the same thing over and over again. Like I found out the hard way, only running lends itself to creating imbalances in other parts of the body, increasing vulnerability to injury.

It is ideal to work on as many movement parameters as possible over the course of time. We might stand, sit, lift, and squat in the course of our daily chores. We might cross-train at the gym and do yoga. We might take walks in the woods, go up and down hills, and step (or leap) over fallen trees. The variability in our daily activities will eventually use our whole bodies, strengthening, supporting, and maintaining our adaptability, and keeping things interesting for us.

Build a Team

It's easy to feel lost and alone when starting something new or when going through a setback due to injury. It's also more difficult to keep going when you feel you're the only one doing it. So, don't be alone!

I'm a huge fan of working with a team of people who support you in your efforts to move. It takes a village to unwind decades of sitting, immobility, bad habits, and injuries, and to finesse new skills and challenges. Your team may simply start with a workout or walking buddy or a yoga or fitness class. You then build it into what you think you need.

Because of a multitude of injuries, my own team is quite substantial and has consisted of many experts coming and going over the years—chiropractors, massage therapists, physical therapists, surgeons (hope you can avoid that one!), trainers, yoga teachers, workout buddies, and podcast creators (for listening to on long hikes). And because progress is a life journey that calls us to step up, have grit, and recover from the discouragement of setbacks, our team includes those who give us solace and support us emotionally—our friends, partners, children, and dogs!

If the professional team concept is new to you, start with bodywork. A skilled massage therapist and chiropractor will support your efforts to release old, negative patterns from the body as you step into your new life of embodiment and increased movement.

Move with Joy

If we don't enjoy the ways we are moving what's the point? Our physiology responds to bad behavior as well as our negative emotions. If we hate what we're doing, it's not worth it, even if it's "good for us." Don't do what you hate. That is not to say that there aren't times when we have to suck it up a bit to do something hard or that pushes us to our limit, or when trying something new that takes us out of our comfort zone. But how do we feel afterward? How do we feel over time as we repeatedly show up for ourselves and as our strength, balance, and function improve?

Do what you enjoy, what you learn to enjoy, or what you believe in. Focus on the performance of your chosen activity and how you feel when you do it and when it's done. Observe what happens to your level of function and wellbeing as your skill and proficiency improve over time. Don't make the mistake of focusing solely on biomarkers or measurements of improved health—like blood pressure, lipid levels, blood sugar, weight or waist measurement. While these measurements have meaning, they are not what sustains our actions. Joy is. So choose what makes you happy and keep at it.

Moving When You Are Persistently Ill, Fatigued, or Debilitated

For some the idea of moving vigorously, or at all, feels overwhelming, and perhaps impossible. No problem. We can gain energy and function by varying our postures, or adding loads in novel ways, whether you can actively move much or not. Try these:

- Walk slowly and mindfully, in bare feet, to your tolerance level. Repeat throughout the day as you can.

- Shift your lying position as often as possible. Challenge yourself with positions you may not normally use, such as front lying, perhaps with upper body bent up, resting on elbows—a good position to read or write for short intervals.

- Try seated positions on the floor: cross-legged, side lying, with pillows, without pillows.

- Try novel or non-uniform surfaces to load and stimulate body parts in new and different ways. For example, roll the bottoms of your feet out on a tennis ball, or stand/rest your feet on a pebble mat or similar textured surface.

- Roll out all of your muscle groups on a foam roller.

- Receive bodywork: massage, chiropractic, physical therapy. These all introduce forces that help mobilize muscles, stimulate circulation, and improve cellular energy production.

Mind-Body Movement: Active Imagination

In addition to actual movement, consider *imagining* yourself moving. By actively visualizing movement, we induce neuroplastic changes in the brain (neuroplasticity is our brains' potential to develop both structurally and functionally) that lead to enhanced physical mass, strength, and function. Athletes and musicians employ this technique, known as active imagination, to improve performance. It has also benefited people unable to move due to paralysis or neurodegenerative disorders. Actively imagining movement of the affected limb—or the entire body—leads to measurable improvements in strength and function.

Exercise: Move Your Body with Your Mind

If you are experiencing a period of enforced immobility, spend time imagining yourself performing the movement of your choice. What you imagine yourself doing will activate neuroplasticity by recruiting dormant movement-related parts of your brain, increasing blood flow to your brain, and strengthening your brain's connections with the rest of your body. Activated neuroplasticity leads to improved strength and function.

Have a specific movement goal in mind, like hiking on your favorite trail in the woods. Be there. See yourself clearly in your mind, fully mobile and enjoying your hike. Hold onto that scene as if it is happening at this very moment and include as much detail as possible, engaging all of your senses. What are you wearing and how do those clothes feel on your body? Who are you with? Feel the breeze against your skin. Hear the leaves rustle and the birds singing. See the deer and squirrels. Smell the dirt and the flowers. Feel the

HEAL KARYN SHANKS MD

uneven surface of the trail and the effort in your thighs as you climb those hills. How do
you feel—what emotions are you experiencing?

Spend fifteen to twenty minutes twice daily with this active visualization practice.
Include as many other scenarios as you would like to deeply activate your brain, support it
as it forms new connections with the rest of your body, and improve your mobility.

Address Injuries

It's important to realize that the vast majority of our musculoskeletal injuries are not problems with the body part per se, but rather problems with our behavior. So, instead of blaming my hamstrings for the chronic pain I feel in them when I sit for prolonged periods of time, I must claim responsibility for my behavior that led to the chronic hamstring injuries in the first place. The fix may well include therapeutic modalities directly to the hamstrings, but it must also include changing movement patterns. For me, this includes less sitting and more variation in movement. For many problems, this may take a team of consultants to figure out. It will require persistence and work. It will always result in global improvements in strength and health that were not necessarily planned for, as you address the root cause.

THE KEY IS TO START—SOMEWHERE, ANYWHERE

If you find yourself stuck and not knowing where to start or how to continue, I have a few recommendations for you.

Remember the power of three we talked about in chapter two? A similar approach keeps your strategy simple (the brain prefers simplicity over multi-tasking) by starting with just three things, while engaging the power of your brain (it loves the number three) to make this whole movement thing happen successfully. Utilizing the power of three may mean taking a big goal and breaking it into three parts to work on every day. It may also mean choosing three ways to add more movement to your life. For instance: begin using a standing desk for part of your workday, spend more time each day in bare feet, and enlist the help of a friend to become your daily walking buddy.

Consider these:

- Keep your plan simple and nonthreatening. Choose something you are likely to succeed at to get yourself started.

- Buddy up. Working out with a friend inspires accountability and makes it more fun.

- Reflect on your barriers to change. Are old stories keeping you from moving forward? Check out chapter eight.

- Hire a fitness trainer or join a class with a professional leader—group fitness, yoga, dance, swimming or water aerobics, or other class of your choice.

- Commit to working with your trainer or group at least two days per week in the beginning. Put this on your calendar and make it nonnegotiable.

LAST THOUGHTS

And finally, move. Move all day. Move with purpose. Move with joy. Move from your strong center. Claim your power. Get yourself ready for what comes next in chapter seven, Nourish, which explores how we nourish our movement and our power through food!

Chapter Seven

NOURISH

Eat for Vitality

Nature, in her great wisdom, provides us with all that we need. In the air, the soil, the plants, and living creatures of this earth. Therein lie the molecules of our lives— our structure, function, energy. Us.

No longer does our culture prepare us for this bounty. No longer is she revered for her perfect match to our needs. We must reclaim this wisdom for ourselves and use it in our lives to nourish, heal, and recover our energy.

WE LITERALLY *ARE* WHAT WE EAT

"Let food be thy medicine and medicine be thy food."

—*Hippocrates*

Grandma was so right: "We are what we eat." Even without reading Hippocrates, she knew. Haven't we heard this a million times? Its repetition has obscured its true meaning, but it's true in a literal way. We *are* what we eat. It's biological fact. The constituents of our food—each individual protein, fat, carbohydrate, and molecule we ingest—become *our* proteins, fats, carbohydrates, and molecules. They become us in the most real, concrete, and certain way. We can label the carbon atoms in the breakfast we eat this morning and see those very same atoms in our brain tissue the next day! Yes, thank you, Grandma, you knew it all along.

Food provides us with the building blocks and chemistry for what makes us who and what we are. You want to build a house? Gotta have the right materials and tools, right? And nothing can be missing, or you're in trouble. Neglect a beam or a few nails? Yikes. Our bodies need the same level of care and attention to detail as the house we're building. We've got to have all the right materials and tools—nutritious food, special nutrients to address unique needs, good eating habits, healthy digestion, and avoidance of food irritants and toxins. We cannot heal, optimize our body's ability to make energy, and run its daily business without these essential nutritional fundamentals.

And though it's certainly molecularly critical for our biology, food has importance that goes beyond that. Food is a rich part of us—the mental, emotional, and spiritual us.

Food is powerful at the cellular level. It is powerful at the level of the person. And it is powerful at the level of the community. We express love and share our sense of community with one another through the preparation and sharing of food. We sit down to meals together as families and communities. We break bread and share wine. Food experienced in these ways elevates its value to us.

We use food to provide comfort and ease suffering. We bring food to those who are grieving, suffering, or hungry. We likewise use food to celebrate life's milestones and sacred passages: birthdays, anniversaries, births, deaths, and life transformations.

Because our food becomes us, it is the foundation for all domains of our health, driving energy, wellbeing, and our potential as human beings. As you'll see, it's not only our essential fuel, it's a critical messenger that changes and controls our biology and determines the expression of our genes. We tend to take our food for granted, caring only about flavors and textures. Though these sensory pleasures of food are important, understanding the role of food in our biology and learning how to eat to optimize function are powerful points of control over our lives.

There isn't a single person who comes to see me who doesn't benefit from a nutrient-dense food plan as part of their energy recovery plan. Even those who stop by for "tweaking" or health optimization, who perhaps don't perceive they have a problem at all, dramatically enhance their energy, clarity, and wellbeing by eating better. They all say they feel "lighter," "happier," and "more like themselves." Their bloat goes away. They shed those unwanted pounds of nagging belly fat. They wake up in the morning with more enthusiasm for what the day will bring.

Think I'm overstating things? Come meet just a couple of my clients and hear their stories.

Joy

Joy came to see me for help after years of persistent fatigue and severe back pain. At age fifty-two, after enduring a lifetime of escalating health problems without solutions, she had just about given up hope. She'd consulted with many medical specialists over the years and received countless therapies that did not work—including drug and surgical interventions that added to her suffering. Most debilitating was the constant back pain, decreased mobility, fatigue, and depression.

She decided to consult with me as a last-ditch effort. After listening to her story, it was clear she had long-standing health issues that were contributing to her current situation. Although each one of these had been addressed by her doctors as discrete, unrelated issues, they were, in fact, a series of dysfunctions, one begetting the next, and escalating into all of her troubles.

After years of antibiotic treatments, anti-inflammatory drugs, and a nutrient-poor standard American diet, her gut lining was damaged, her immune system was persistently activated, her gut flora—the billions of microorganisims inhabiting her gut, central to good health—was imbalanced. She was severely malnourished (yes, even in middle-class America!). These issues served as the genesis of the systemic inflammation that was contributing to her pain and fatigue.

We decided to start her treatment with the basics: a nutrient-dense food plan that would remove the foods she was sensitive to, heal her gut, and reduce inflammation. Initially she felt a bit daunted by the number of foods I recommended she eliminate, so we eased her into the plan instead, working first with the most common food irritant suspects: strict elimination of gluten, cow's milk, processed grains, and sugar for a one-month trial. We added some nutrients to help her gut heal, reduce inflammation, and support her gut flora.

To our delight, when she returned in one month, she had experienced complete resolution of all back pain. Her energy was soaring, her head was clear, and her headaches were gone. She felt like a new woman. Repeat lab work showed normalized thyroid tests and inflammatory markers, both mildly abnormal before she started her food and nutrition plan. Because of the dramatic nature of her response to these relatively simple interventions, she was highly motivated to continue them for life.

Joy was amazed at the change that was possible. But I wasn't. Joy's is not an unusual story at all. I frequently work with people who have become sick from the damage caused to their guts by antibiotics and anti-inflammatory drugs (both used cavalierly in our culture), who go on to develop gut-related dysfunction (often referred to as "irritable bowel syndrome") and activation of their immune systems (manifesting as everything from asthma, allergies, autoimmune problems, to brain and mood dysfunction).

Joy's journey was compounded by inadequate nutrient intake that is an inevitable part of eating the standard American diet. So, although the result of fixing things was profound, the fix, itself, was easy—eating healthy food, eliminating food irritants, optimizing nutrition guided by comprehensive nutrition testing, rebuilding of the gut flora, and taking inflammation-modulating supplements.

Joy's story is all about the power of food, particularly how a commonly practiced American lifestyle can lead to such widespread systemic inflammation with a multitude of debilitating problems.

Gary

Some folks need more intensive food plans to heal. Gary came to see me when he was sixty-four years old and had suffered from severe joint and muscle pain for decades. The pain was diffuse but seemed to concentrate along his spine and sacroiliac joints. Over the years he had been diagnosed with multiple autoimmune disorders—destructive disorders brought about by immune cells persistently activated against one's own tissue, rather than against invading microbes or allergens—including sarcoidosis, ankylosing spondylitis, autoimmune thyroiditis, and celiac disease. He also had kidney and liver damage from the destructive inflammation in his body.

HEAL KARYN SHANKS MD

He'd followed all the instructions provided to him by his various doctors and subspecialists over the years, including taking immune suppressive drugs to reduce inflammation, but he still felt bad. He was tired of throwing drugs at the problems when they clearly were not helping. Most important to him, his energy was very low, he was short of breath, and he felt depressed. He had retired early due to his illness and was trying to find a better way in his life. What he really wanted was to be out of pain and happy again.

Although his journey to recovery took some unexpected twists and turns before we made significant headway, the basics were the same: remove sources of inflammation, heal the damage, prevent future inflammation. We put him on the Gut-Immune Restoration Intensive Nutrition (GRIN) food plan (details later in this chapter), an intensive autoimmune food plan, which heals the gut and reduces inflammation. These measures helped, but he continued to have a very stiff spine, and sore hands and sacroiliac joints, making it hard to move around. We discovered that he had some unexpected food sensitivities. He'd been using coconut products extensively as a source of healthy fat in his diet. Taking these out reduced his pain and improved his energy. He was also "cheating" with coffee regularly, which wasn't allowed on his food plan. Once he stopped ingesting both coffee and coconut products, he experienced complete resolution of back pain and his hands were much better. The extensive erosive osteoarthritis in his hands put him at a mechanical disadvantage, but he was quite happy with the improvement.

Of course, we also had him optimize nutrition and provide extra support for parts of his systems biology that were particularly challenged by his years of illness—especially adrenal function, gut, and detoxification. To our delight his kidney and liver tests all improved, in addition to his improved energy, wellbeing, and overall function.

Food Is Information

We live in two worlds: the inner world of our physical bodies and the outer world of the space our bodies move through. These inner and outer worlds are in constant communication through our senses of sight, smell, touch, and so on, sending messages about what's going on. Our food is also an unsung messenger communicating with our inner world. It not only tells our bodies things like when food is plentiful (time to build stores of fat) or scarce (time to shift to a ketone-based energy supply), but also signals changes in our body's chemistry and function on a moment by moment basis.

The Sugar-Fatigue Story

Ever have that post-meal energy drop? Wonder why?

Well, it goes like this. We eat a carbohydrate-rich meal (breakfast Danish, bagels, sandwich for lunch), which is all digested promptly into sugar. Toxic to our cells and tissues in excess, the sugar in our blood must be reckoned with immediately. That very sugar from our food sends signals to our body to produce insulin. Insulin communicates with our cells to move that sugar from our blood, convert it to glycogen or fat, and store it for future use. Our blood insulin levels rise, but the process lags a bit (it takes some time to produce and distribute it). So, the meal is over, the excess sugar has been stored, but the insulin level is still high. This drives more sugar out of the blood and into the cells, lowering blood sugar levels further. The drop in our blood sugar makes us feel tired, causing us to reach for that afternoon cup of coffee we really don't need. The blood sugar drop signals our brains that a critical energy source may be plummeting. Is this a crisis? Ensuing famine? The brain sounds the alarm, initiating stress hormone release to support energy and survival. This explains the anxious, jittery, spacey feeling that can follow a sugary or high-carb meal.

This is a simplification of a complicated process, but it gives you an idea of how food is a messenger delivering information that starts a whole cascade of signals and events that control our bodies, affecting not just the microscopic physiology that we don't feel but also the physical and mental effects that we do. It's doing what our biology evolved to do. That post-high-carb-meal fatigue is an expected biological adaptation. The lesson for us is to understand the context of the message—to consume less sugar and high-sugar-content-carbohydrate foods.

Food Becomes Our Internal Systems Biology

Our genes and every one of our trillions of cells, including the genes and cells of our gut flora, are in constant conversation with our food. Every molecule we ingest has something very specific to communicate to our bodies, becoming our internal systems biology. Food becomes all the important processes that keep us alive and help us thrive: energy production, detoxification, gut function, microbiome health, immune and inflammatory function, adaptable stress response, structure and movement, hormones and communication, and healthy brain and nervous system.

Bottom line? If we eat healthy food, the messages delivered to our internal biology are positive and support good health and optimal function. If we do not eat well, or if we eat in ways that are incompatible with our needs, then the messages delivered do not support good health, leading to loss of function and suffering.

WE'RE MALNOURISHED AND TOXIC

It's obvious why food should be so important to our lives, so why do we have a problem?

We're Disconnected from Our Food

In the Western world, we've become disconnected from our food. It has become industrialized, processed, fast, and no longer the product of our gardens and kitchens. That isn't a bad thing by definition. One of the key developmental milestones of any culture is when enough of the population is freed up from growing food and meeting subsistence needs to develop other interests such as art and science.

But as we've stepped further away from our own food production, we know less and less about nutrition and food preparation. As a result, we eat increasingly poor diets. We've given the responsibility for deciding what we eat to others and have generally not asked or challenged them about why they make the food choices for us that they do. We blindly accept that something as simple as a loaf of bread should have a long list of ingredients we can't even pronounce. Our culture commoditizes our food, placing greater value on cost and speed of preparation, shelf life, and quick consumer appeal, rather than on nutritional value.

Food is Disconnected from Our Medicine

Furthermore, our medical system does not acknowledge the central role of food in health and healing. Nutrition is inadequately taught in medical schools. A review in the journal of the Association of American Medical Colleges, *Academic Medicine*, found that, "On average, US medical schools offer 19.6 hours of nutrition-related education across four years of medical education. This corresponds to less than one percent of estimated total lecture hours. Moreover, the majority of this educational content relates to biochemistry, not diets or practical, food-related decision-making." As a direct result, food and nutrition do not become central themes within the context of the physician-patient encounter, in spite of food's vital importance to our health. And this contributes to the persistence of a standard Western diet that is harmful.

We Have Higher Nutritional Demands

In addition to our collective food choices, we're increasingly challenged by environmental stresses and toxicities that increase the nutrient requirements of our bodies.

High stress requires high energy—the whole point of stress is to ramp up our bodies' energy producing system to help us engage successfully with our challenges. But energy production is expensive, requiring an enormous array of hormones, enzymes, vitamins, minerals, and cofactors to operate.

Where do these come from? We make them from the food we eat.

Likewise, toxin removal from the body is necessary to sustain life. Detoxification is also energy and nutrient expensive. We've got to support it every day with the nutrients we get from food. Sluggishness in this process, which occurs when nutrient need outweighs supply, is a common problem. A yearly detox program doesn't magically fix everything. Detoxification is a 24/7 proposition that requires healthy protein, fat, vitamins, minerals, and antioxidants from food.

We're Inundated with Bad Food

For all of us, the sheer abundance of food is a modern-day temptation that leads to many health challenges. Our obsession with sugar and processed grain products (which are digested into sugar) may well be the driving force for our exposure to the number one toxin in the Western world today (you guessed it—sugar!), which is responsible for millions of deaths every year and billions—perhaps trillions—in annual healthcare costs.

To complicate things, for many communities there is an abundance of the most nutrient-poor and toxic foods (high sugar content, overly processed), while fresh, nutritious, plant-based foods are scarce. This encourages poor food choices even when the desire to eat better is there. It's also true that premium food is the most expensive, making a good diet harder to attain for disadvantaged communities. Processed boxed grain-based carbohydrates are cheap, while fresh fruits and vegetables cost more. Organic foods are simply not affordable for many Americans. The healthiest sources of animal meat products—those that are raised in the pasture, eating only what they need, free to graze on their native food sources without the stress of industrialized feed lots—are relatively expensive, while industrialized meat—raised in crowded conditions, overfed and fattened by foods they can't digest, often treated with cruelty—is cheap and readily available.

A lot of this is a cultural problem that we're beginning to address as a society. But we also need to address it at the individual level, with individuals accepting responsibility for their food choices and the know-how needed to prepare fresh healthy food. If we have more to spend on the big TV, but we feel sluggish and depressed and our joints hurt because we're eating poorly, are we better off? I can't tell you how much of your income is right for you to spend on food or how much of your time and energy should be devoted to cooking. But, if you ever find yourself saying it's too costly or inconvenient to eat well, then ask yourself: How much is your health worth? How much is it worth to feel really good? To feel that you have unlimited potential? To feel like yourself again?

Ugh—Sugar! (Sugar Is a Toxin)

In excess, sugar is as toxic as any environmental chemical that we are exposed to. In fact, it has become the most ubiquitous and harmful toxin known to mankind due to its abundance and massive consumption by people worldwide. It is not an essential human nutrient. Our bodies don't require the simple sugars found in table sugar, honey, or plant syrups. Still, the average American consumes about one hundred thirty pounds of sugar per year, mostly in the form of soft drinks sweetened with high fructose corn syrup (HFCS), sugar additives, candy, baked goods, and fruit drinks.

While all sugar is bad in excess, including the sugar derived from "natural" sources such as honey, agave, maple syrup, fruit, and starchy vegetables, the biggest villain in the sugar pantheon is high fructose corn syrup (HFCS). It does not require digestion, therefore is freely absorbed, rapidly making its way to the liver, where it is quickly converted to fat. There is no hormonal feedback associated with its consumption to control intake, so large quantities can be consumed without the usual signaling that alerts us about having had enough. Regular intake of HFCS leads to obesity and fatty liver, one of the number one causes of liver failure in the Western world.

Because sugar is so toxic to our bodies, a great deal of physiological energy goes into keeping our blood levels in a safe range. Glucose in excess gloms onto all our structural proteins and changes their function. This is how the devastating end-organ complications of long-standing diabetes evolve. Proteins altered by sugar are referred to as "advanced glycosolyation end-products" (AGEs). These structurally and functionally damaged proteins are recognized by our immune cells as foreign, driving a full-on immune response. This is how eating sugar drives the inflammatory storm that causes so much destruction and dysfunction.

High blood sugar and its most severe expression, diabetes, results in catastrophic health consequences: vascular disease leading to heart attack, stroke, and organ failure; retinal damage leading to vision loss; kidney disease and high blood pressure; dementia and neurodegenerative disorders; painful neuropathy; obesity; inflammatory disorders; liver disease; and cancers.

Grains Are Sugar

Grain that has been pulverized to create flour products used in breads, cereals, crackers, and other food products are digested very rapidly into sugar and absorbed into the body as such. The glycemic index (the rate and amount of sugar made available to the body by the food in comparison to table sugar, sucrose) is actually higher for processed grains than for table sugar. In addition, most modern grains have been extensively genetically altered to increase their carbohydrate content. So even "healthy" whole grains have high sugar contents, joining the ranks of toxic foods.

Sugar Addiction

Sugar is *hard* to let go—it's addictive. It's an obsession. We love the way sugar tastes, feels, and what it does to us. We get a little shot of pleasure. Yep, it smacks us right in the pleasure centers of our brains and drags us out of whatever funk or low-energy state we might be in.

Bad news: it's temporary, our bodies don't need it, and it's harmful. It never sustains itself. It always has repercussions. Our blood sugar rises initially and our brain blisses out. But then the crash comes: insulin rises, blood sugar drops, brain goes into spasm, and we feel fatigued, shaky, depressed, and shamed because, well, we did it again. Our dysfunctional relationship with sugar is just not worth it. Sugar makes us a lot of promises and never follows through, leaving us desperate and in the dumps every time.

Letting go of sugar is hard. Join me for an exercise (see appendix A) to transform deprivation into something positive and empowering.

CALL YOUR POWER BACK—YOU CAN CHOOSE

Eating well is hard. But we can do hard things—we've called our power back. We've imagined and articulated our story of healing. We've created space for this. We've called in love. We've found our strong center, and from this place of strength we make all our healing decisions.

We have chosen, as a culture, to value being able to go to the grocery store and buy a can of vegetables and package of chemically altered, industrialized meat, instead of inspecting, selecting, chopping, and preparing our meal ourselves from scratch. We have chosen to go to fast-food restaurants on our way home from work rather than plan and prepare dinner in advance. These choices are not always bad. But they're lifestyle choices. There are consequences. And the choice is a question of balance. Making everything from scratch is not feasible for most families. But eating nothing but processed, nutrient-poor food is not feasible for the body. Going to a fast-food restaurant with hungry kids after a soccer game is great (and I've done it many times), but eating fast food every night is a terrible idea. It's all a question of balance, and always a decision, however consciously or unconsciously those decisions are made.

Realizing it's a choice—calling your power back—is the first step to reconnecting to your food. You can decide what and how to eat. You can choose to learn how to cook one simple healthy thing from scratch each week and build on that. Many will say they don't have time for that. But remember the story of not enough time? It's always an excuse. We've created space, let go of distractions, and reclaimed time. This space and time is perfect for now adding healthy food to our lives. But no one expects you to suddenly start growing and preparing all your food. Starting with baby steps (remember, just three small things), we can all become more conscious and thoughtful about how and what we eat. I'm here to help.

BUILDING A FOOD PLAN

It's hard to say what the specifics of any one person's food plan should be without knowing them. For our food plans to work for us as individuals, they must address our unique needs as well as our likes and dislikes. Asking someone to switch to a diet they can't stand eating is not going to work. So, while you will have to tailor each of these suggested plans to your own circumstances, here are the two core food plans I teach to my own clients. The Foundational Intensive Nutrition Energy (FINE) food plan is my core basic starting point for nutritious eating. It's likely the plan you'll want to try first. It emphasizes core nutritional principles while addressing inflammation. My more intensive food plan, the Gut-Immune Restoration Intensive Nutrition (GRIN) food plan is a "next step" plan, addressing more advanced gut, brain, inflammatory, and autoimmune conditions.

Before we go into the specifics of each plan, let's explore some general tips for developing and sticking to a food plan.

Food Sensitivities and Intolerances

Food sensitivities and intolerances are commonplace and play an important role in how we structure personalized food plans. First of all, how do you know if you have food sensitivities or intolerances? These can manifest as any adverse reaction that relates directly back to the food you consume.

Food allergies could be considered sensitivities, though they are not the same thing. Allergies involve a highly specific type of immune cell reaction to food proteins, resulting in very characteristic symptoms. Specific sensitized immune cells, upon exposure to a food allergen, immediately release chemical inflammation mediators (like histamines, prostaglandins, and leukotrienes) that cause hives, itchy skin, runny nose, sinus congestion, sneezing, headaches, wheezing, shortness of breath, abdominal pain, fast heart rate, and anxiety. On the more severe end of the spectrum of these symptoms is anaphylaxis—when the reaction is so severe that airways are compromised, and one may experience life-threatening trouble with breathing and control over cardiovascular system responses. These require emergency treatment at home (EpiPen, anti-histamines) or the emergency room.

Food sensitivities and intolerances are not the same as allergies. They do not have the potential for sudden life-threatening symptoms as allergies do, though they can still cause great suffering due to the inflammation, tissue damage, pain, and hormonal and brain chemistry imbalances they can cause.

Common Food Sensitivities and Intolerances

- Food proteins that trigger a "delayed type" hypersensitivity response by immune cells lining the gut: such as gluten, grains, animal milk protein, eggs.

- Foods that may not digest well (even when digestion itself is functioning well), leading to gut discomfort, gas, bloating, and diarrhea; foods with high contents of poorly absorbed carbohydrates referred to by the acronym, FODMAPs (fermentable oligo-, di-, mono-saccharides, and polyols). These include fructose and fructans, galactooligosaccharides, disaccharides (lactose), monosaccharides (fructose), and sugar alcohols (polyols—sorbitol, mannitol, xylitol, maltitol).

- Naturally occurring food chemicals that are irritating and may be difficult to remove in predisposed individuals: such as tyramines and histamines (found in aged and fermented foods); and oxalates, alkaloids, and lectins (found in many plant foods).

- Foods that irritate the gut lining, leading to increases in gut permeability, increased systemic toxicity, and inflammation: such as grains, cow's milk, eggs, beans and legumes, nightshades, nuts.

- Processed foods with high sugar content: grains, fructose, high-fructose corn syrup, sucrose, all sugars.

- Food additives and toxins: contaminants (pesticides, herbicides, heavy metals), dyes and coloring agents, gums, damaged fats (hydrogenated, trans, or rancid fats), charred meat.

Reversing Food Sensitivities and Intolerances

If you believe you have been suffering from the effects of food sensitivities and intolerances, it will be important to follow a food plan with one hundred percent strictness. Both of the food plans that I will lay out will exclude common inflammation triggers, though the GRIN plan will do so more thoroughly.

It is imperative to allow ample time to reverse the irritant and inflammatory processes responsible for causing the damage, and for healing to take place. With food sensitivities, the inflammatory response to culprit foods occurs with the same vigorousness to a very small amount of the food as it does to a large quantity due to the protective sensitizing nature of the immune cells (they know that even very small quantities of some irritants are dangerous). Simply reducing the quantity, but not completely eliminating the culprit food will not help, and often make symptoms worse.

If you have true immunological sensitivities to food, you may feel worse before you feel better once you've implemented the FINE or GRIN food plans. Your immune system remains vigilant as your body becomes accustomed to the absence of the culprit foods. This lasts just a few days to a week or so. Expect it so you will not be surprised. Treat yourself symptomatically, just as you would if you had the flu. And remember, *this too shall pass.*

Systemic Inflammatory Conditions and Autoimmunity

For many people food sensitivities are part of a constellation of system-wide symptoms and problems caused by inflammation, impaired gut permeability, and autoimmunity. The FINE food plan may be a good starting place; however, it is possible that you will need to use a more aggressive strategy for a period of time. These details are outlined later in this chapter, in the section, Gut-Immune Restoration Intensive Nutrition (GRIN) food plan.

Metabolic Syndrome (Blood Sugar and Insulin Regulation Problems)

Metabolic syndrome is a group of conditions with shared physiology that often occur together, including high blood pressure, high blood sugar, and excess belly fat. For those who have metabolic syndrome symptoms, it's ideal to follow a food plan strictly. Many of the restricted foods, such as grains (even healthy whole grains) release large amounts of sugar when digested. This leads to excess insulin release in the body. When persistent, this will induce a stress response, inflammation, increased belly fat, and a whole host of "downstream" problems that are part of the metabolic syndrome physiology.

For Vegans and Vegetarians

My food plans will be a challenge for vegetarians and vegans in the protein and complete nutrition departments. Without animal flesh, fish, dairy products, eggs, beans, or legumes as protein sources, you will have to be much more mindful of the protein content of the foods that you eat. You will likely need to incorporate healthy protein supplements into your diet, particularly if you are active.[20] Several important nutrients can only be obtained from animal products in levels that are adequate to support optimal health (vitamin B12, choline, omega-3 fatty acids, many minerals, iron, and vitamin D). Consider

----

[20] See Karyn Shanks MD. *How to Optimize Protein for Energy and Vitality*. 2019: karynshanksmd.com/2019/08/16/optimal-protein-energy-vitality/

working with a trusted health practitioner or functional nutrition specialist well versed in this style of eating.

Your Challenge

Success starts with a decision—a commitment. I challenge you to commit to six weeks of complete strictness to your chosen food plan. Keep a food journal and carefully document your food and liquid intake as well as any symptoms. If you experience symptoms, such as pain, fatigue, or brain fog, rate them daily on a scale of zero to ten. Observe the change.

Once the six-week introduction period is over, if you decide to stray, do so mindfully. Choose your "off-plan" food carefully, eat it joyfully, and document what you did so you can observe the consequences. Many food sensitivity-related symptoms don't occur right away, but as long as several days later.

If you are not able to achieve a six-week trial at this time, you may benefit from shorter periods. In general, it takes six to twelve weeks to correct the immune and hormonal responses that cause symptoms. However, in just two weeks (shorter periods than two weeks may not allow you to get over the initial period of not feeling well) you may get to experience some of the benefits of eating more nutritious and less toxic food.

Remember, many people feel worse before they feel better, especially those who are making a dramatic overhaul of their usual eating plan. This will last a few days up to a few weeks. Track your symptoms carefully and hang in there. If you are concerned, talk to your trusted healthcare provider before giving up.

Common Challenges and Pitfalls for Beginners Adopting a Food Plan

Adopting a healthier eating strategy absolutely will challenge you. Change is always a challenge. For some of you there may be a period of intense deprivation and perhaps withdrawal-like symptoms as you move away from your current way of eating. You may need to learn a whole new way of eating, cooking, shopping, socializing, eating out, and traveling. People may be curious or downright critical as you break away from the usual routine. Embrace these challenges. Understand where you are headed. Carefully observe the changes that occur as your health improves. Seek out wise counsel and support for getting through the rough patches.

Feeling Deprived

We derive pleasure and nourishment from our bad habits and favorite foods—Why else would we eat them? It's hard to voluntarily let go of the intense—though short lived—benefits of our favorite comfort foods. Sugar, grains, and cow's milk can cause real physical addiction. It's not uncommon to crave them for several days up to a couple of weeks after eliminating them from your diet.[21]

Physical Symptoms

Again, expect to feel worse before you feel better if you are making serious changes, especially with sugar and foods that commonly cause sensitivities, as well as sugar. Fatigue, headaches, lack of motivation, weakness, sleepiness, foggy head, intense cravings—even flu-like symptoms—are all fair game. They will last just a few days up to a week or two. Rest, adequate hydration, and ample "allowed" food intake will all help. Some find relief with the use of OTC activated charcoal, which soaks up some of the immune cell chemicals that cause many of these symptoms—two capsules between meals as needed.

Organization

This is key, and what most of my clients struggle with the most in the early phase of the FINE and GRIN food plans. Learn the food plan first. Then plan your meals and snacks ahead of time so your pantry and fridge are well stocked with everything you need when you need it. I swear, you'll get good at this!

---

[21] Work with my deprivation-busting mindfulness practice in appendix A: Deprivation: How to Cope.

Not Eating Enough

Some people start out on this plan and do not eat enough in the early stages while they are learning. They often lose weight quickly and feel hungry, tired, and weak. This is easily remedied by careful planning so that ample food is available for all meals and snacks.

Social Gatherings and Eating Out

It is very hard to stick to this plan at the majority of restaurants, especially chains and fast-food restaurants, and at social gatherings where the other participants don't eat the way you do now. In the beginning it is best to work on learning the fundamentals of the food plan and food preparation by eating at home. Once you are good at this, you will know how to select restaurants and know what questions to ask your server regarding ingredients you are trying to avoid. For social gatherings, you may need to eat beforehand or take your own food. Your close friends will get to know your new sensibilities about food, so tell them what you can't eat and offer to bring a dish.

Travel

You will need to get savvy about how to have your needs met while away from home. This may include planning ahead to find grocery stores and restaurants that can accommodate your food plan, packing and transporting food, taking healthy meal replacement products such as bars and protein supplements, or planning for accommodations where you can have a kitchen and do your own cooking. This gets tricky, but it's something you will become good at over time.

Getting Frustrated and Giving Up

This may be due to the challenges of making change or getting organized around new skills and habits. It may also be related to feeling poorly in the early stages. It is good to know what to expect and to prepare yourself for what is to come. Read this section thoroughly and create a careful plan for yourself. Remember that failure is your best teacher. If you fall, get back up.

Family and Friend Backlash and Lack of Support

People close to you may not understand your efforts to change your diet. Some may even try to sabotage your efforts at self-improvement. Or perhaps they don't understand and feel just as overwhelmed as you do. Share your educational materials with them and don't forget to *ask* for help! In the end, this is your life, your self-care, and only you can decide what is best for you.

Let Go of the Need to Be "All Ready"

We've talked about this before: don't wait to begin until you're "all ready." When are we ever ready—*really* ready—to step into change and into our fears about what may happen next, about how hard or impossible it all seems? Sure, it helps to make a plan and get organized, but we may never possess that deep sense in our guts that now is the time. However, in spite of not *feeling* ready, we all have the capacity to be brave, uncertain, and unsure about the outcome and still move forward. We can make the decision and step into action.

No Calorie Counting

Follow the simple rules for eating in these food plans, and there will be no need to count calories. Eat your fill and enjoy what you eat. You will find that you will be less hungry during the day and eat less overall. In addition, once you have completely eliminated grains (particularly wheat) and sugar, you will no longer have the addictive relationship with food that leads to compulsive eating and unstable mood and energy throughout the day. What liberation. That is not to say that calories don't factor into our ultimate strategy. Clearly eating calories in excess of our needs will put a stop to needed fat loss. Eating a bagful of those healthy, high fat, high calorie nuts is probably not a good idea. However, for now, as you learn, calorie counting is not necessary.

Also, please stay off the scale during the first six weeks while you are incorporating this food plan into your life. I want your focus and emphasis to be on the *quality* of food you are eating and the lifestyle change involved in making this happen. Your weight is not the central issue. It is a side effect of how you are eating and the condition of your health.

Weight loss is inevitable on both the FINE and GRIN food plans. Please focus on learning and get away from obsessing about your weight.

FINE—THE FOUNDATIONAL INTENSIVE NUTRITION ENERGY FOOD PLAN (A *REAL FOOD* PLAN)

"Eat (real) food. Not too much. Mostly plants."

—*Michael Pollan, Food Rules*

In some ways this food plan is about going back to our roots. It's about eating real food, grown in favorable conditions, prepared simply and deliciously, shared with those we love, eaten slowly, and just enough to meet our needs.

But it's also about moving forward in our age of high technology and convenience and using the positive attributes of our modern age as an asset to improve our nutrition and ability to use food for healing. It is not about trying to mimic what we think our ancestors were doing, but more about evolution and optimizing what we have available to us for our own benefit.

The FINE food plan provides intensive nutrition to support all of our body's needs while eliminating foods that cause inflammation, toxicity, elevated blood sugar levels, and damage to our metabolism. Those who eat this way get to enjoy robust energy, reversal of inflammatory conditions, clearer thinking, attainment of ideal body weight, and more joyful lives.

FINE Is Not a Paleo or Ancestral Diet (Strictly Speaking)

The FINE food plan I teach is *not* a Paleo or "ancestral" diet. Paleo is a cultural movement that seeks to fundamentally change how people eat, and it has great intentions: to improve the quality of what people eat by borrowing from the heritage of our ancestors. There are elements that are of great value and have provided tremendous inspiration for how I think about food and what I recommend to my clients. There are also elements within the Paleo movement that are misguided.

The emphasis on eating real food and more plants by some versions of the modern Paleo diet is good. Encouraging persistent overconsumption of animal products and repetitive food groups without regard to nutritional diversity, seasonal changes, and personal preferences is not good. Moreover, our Paleolithic ancestors roamed the earth before the time of agriculture: they foraged, hunted, and to a limited extent, grew their food. Tribes all over the world adapted to their unique habitats and had greatly different diets as a result. Their lifestyles were completely different than our own not only in terms of types of foods consumed, but movement, relationships, and stressors. Being dogmatic about protocols and strategies fit for *everyone* does not take into consideration our individual differences and preferences.

But our bodies—our genetics and physiologies—did, in fact, arise from our ancestors. And these haven't changed. We can take lessons from what we know about them. They ate real food, they seldom consumed in excess of their needs, they moved their bodies a lot, and they lived in closely-knit communities. These are the positive attributes of Paleolithic cultures that we can capitalize on.

The FINE Food Plan is Founded on the Principles of the Healthiest Eating

- Nutrient-rich (macronutrients—protein and fat, micronutrients, antioxidants, phytonutrients);

- Avoids common food toxins and irritants;

- Supports the microbiome;

- Optimizes the gut-immune environment.

The FINE Food Plan Is Simple

- Eat real food only and always.

- Avoid all processed, refined, or altered (other than cooking or blending) foods.

- Avoid all sugars (most of the time), aside from those occurring naturally in healthy plant foods (we'll get into what "healthy" is in a bit).

- Eat healthy fat.

- Eat enough healthy protein to meet your needs.

- Eat mostly plants.

- Eat a variety of plants of many colors.

- Feed your microbiome (the microorganisms that share your body with you!).

- Eat fresh food, farm-to-table, seasonably.

- Eat mindfully, joyfully, and socially.

- Don't overeat.

Foods to *Include* in Your FINE Food Plan

Healthy meat choices, eggs, and fish

Eat only grass-fed beef options, free-range poultry and eggs, wild game, and wild-caught fatty fish such as salmon, herring and sardines.

Use organ meat from pasture-raised animal. Include protein in every meal and refer to the protein counter on my website to determine your total daily protein needs and plan your meals and snacks accordingly.[22] Most people will need four to six ounces—approximately the size of a deck of cards—of protein at a meal to meet their protein requirements.

——————————————————

[22] Karyn Shanks, MD. See *How to Optimize Protein for Energy and Vitality.* 2019: karynshanksmd.com/2019/08/16/optimal-protein-energy-vitality/

Non-Starchy Vegetables

Eat mostly greens but make sure to include a multitude of other colors. Eat dark-green leafy vegetables daily—spinach, kale, collard, arugula, chard.

Emphasize the crucifer family: cabbage, kale, broccoli, broccoli sprouts, and Brussels sprouts. Include garlic and onions liberally.

Minimize starchy vegetables such as carrots, yams, and potatoes but do include them in small quantities, as they are rich in nutrition.

A simple guideline for quantity is that veggies should take up two-thirds of your plate at each meal, or eight to twelve cups total (when raw—note that steamed and sautéed vegetables will shrink considerably).

Those with metabolic syndrome (high blood pressure, high blood sugar, diabetes, vascular disease, or obesity): avoid starchy veggies altogether!

Low Sugar-Content Fruit

Eat mostly berries (blueberries, raspberries, blackberries, and so on), and may include apples and pears. Pomegranates and cranberries are good options. Save sweeter fruits (e.g. peaches, bananas, apples, pineapple) for special treats and desserts.

Those with metabolic syndrome: avoid all fruit other than berries, tart apples, cranberries and pomegranates.

Nuts and seeds

Stick to raw, fresh options and avoid peanuts (these are actually legumes and can promote inflammation). Roasting can damage the fats in many nuts, making them more toxic.

Nuts and seeds contain healthy fats, which are vital to our good health; however be aware of their high calorie content to avoid over-consumption. Ground flax and hemp seeds and whole chia seeds provide a lot of fiber, protein, and healthy fats—include these daily. They mix well in smoothies.

Bone Broth

Make bone broth from the leftover bones of free-range chickens, grass-fed beef, or game. Include it in soups and stews, sauté vegetables with it, or drink it by itself. You may add beef-derived collagen hydrosylate (see below) to increase protein content and make a substantial meal or snack out of it. Plus, your dog will love you for adding bone broth to his/her food!

Spices, Condiments, Food Supplements

Some of my favorite highly nutritive varieties of spices and flavoring agents are cinnamon, turmeric, cayenne, cardamom, black pepper, paprika, ginger, rosemary, thyme, basil, sencha ground green tea, vegetable proteins (such as hemp and pea proteins), gelatin or hydrolyzed collagen derived from grass-fed cows (to use as a protein supplement).

Healthy Fats

Coconut oil and coconut milk: For coconut milk, use the full-fat culinary version sold in cans or make your own. Avoid the diluted version of coconut milk sold in cartons. Make sure your coconut milk and oil are organically sourced. The fats in coconut are rich in medium-chain triglycerides, important for structure and energy production. They are also rich in fats (lauric acid, caprylic acid, capric acid) that may have important antimicrobial effects.

Avocados and Avocado oil: These contain potent antioxidants known as carotenoids, phytosteroids, and polyhydroxylated fatty alcohols, all of which help modulate inflammation in the body. The oleic acid in avocados is a monounsaturated fat that reduces the risk of vascular disease.

Olives and Olive Oil: Olive oil is one of the healthiest foods on the planet. Not only is it rich in heart and vasculature-protective monounsaturated fats, but it also contains a diverse array of antioxidant and anti-inflammatory nutrients that have been shown to reduce inflammation, cancer risk, allergies, cardiovascular problems, osteoporosis and more. Buy only organic, unrefined varieties and store in dark containers in cool areas to prevent spoilage. Buy only "extra virgin" or "fresh pressed" varieties.

Omega-3 Fats: (fish oil, algae-derived DHA): These have many health benefits as necessary structural fats for cell membranes and anti-inflammatory molecules. If you don't eat fatty fish like wild-caught salmon regularly, you would benefit from supplementing with a good quality fish oil supplement containing EPA and DHA (the biologically important omega-3 fats).

Beans and Legumes

Use the full spectrum of beans, legumes, lentils, and other split legumes. Limit the amount you consume to keep the sugar content of your diet low. Omit them entirely if you suspect you have food sensitivities.

Teas

You may include unsweetened green tea (preferably Sencha ground green tea powder, which is grown in the sun and higher in antioxidants while lower in caffeine content compared to Macha, which is grown in the shade), black and white tea varieties, rooibos, and all herbal teas in your food plan.

Fermented Foods

Fermented vegetables such as sauerkraut and kimchi are allowed and provide essential probiotic organisms. Kombucha may be consumed in moderation (one half to one cup per day).

Fluids

It is important to stay well hydrated. Most people need a minimum of two quarts of liquid per day. You may use filtered water, mineral water, green tea, herbal tea, and bone broth.

Smoothies

This is a convenient and potentially delicious way to create a meal while on this plan. Simply include only those foods allowed on the plan. Include hydrolyzed collagen as your protein, some fat and water and/or coconut milk to create a meal that includes all major food groups to sustain you through part of your day.

Nutritional Supplements

Most nutritional supplements that have been specifically prescribed for you to meet your unique needs are allowed on the FINE food plan if manufacturers have been careful to exclude the undesirable ingredients. Work with your Functional Medicine practitioner on this if necessary.

Foods to *Avoid* on Your FINE Food Plan

All Grains (wheat, rye, barley, oats, corn, rice)

Grains can be irritants to the immune system as well as the lining of the gastrointestinal tract. All of today's genetically engineered grain varieties are high in sugar content and release excesses of sugar through the digestive process.

Check with your nutrition consultant, but some "pseudograins," such as quinoa and millet, which are actually seeds, may be allowed.

All Animal Milk Products (includes cow, goat, and sheep's milk)

Animal milk is proinflammatory by virtue of its major protein, casein, and one of its predominant fats, arachadonic acid. Casomorphins are produced in the digestive process of milk and behave like opiates that can cause mood and cognitive dysfunction in susceptible individuals.

All Processed, Synthetic Foods, Preservatives and Additives

Most of these are manufactured molecules that displace real food, are void of nutrition, often high in calories, and can be irritants harmful to human health.

Unhealthy Meats

These include commercial corn-fed feedlot beef, commercial poultry and eggs, many farm-raised fish and all large predator fish (such as tuna and swordfish). (The status of farm-raised fish is changing as growers are responding to the need for ethically and nutritionally raised fish. See National Resources Defense Council's, NRDC, website for more information.)

Feedlot beef are treated with the utmost cruelty and are obese, unhealthy animals. Their meat is less nutritious than their pasture-raised counterparts, containing an abundance of unhealthy fats and higher levels of pesticide and antibiotic residues.

Fish not wild-caught as well as larger predator fish are suspect for pesticides or heavy metal contamination. Refer to the NRDC's detailed guide about choosing fish with the lowest mercury content.

Excesses of Sugar

This includes the sugar naturally occurring in fruits and vegetables (sweet fruit and starchy veggies). The literature is now huge on negative health impact of dietary sugars.

Artificial and Non-Nutritive Sweeteners

Avoid all sugar substitutes and artificial sweeteners that add sweetness to food and beverages but have no nutritional value. These include sucralose, Splenda, aspartame and sugar alcohols (such as mannitol, sorbitol, dextrose and xylitol). Stevia and monk fruit may be consumed sparingly—the sweet taste leads to insulin release, promotion of inflammation, and may support sugar addiction.

Unhealthy Fats

Omit all trans or hydrogenated fats, fat from commercial meats, damaged fats found in rancid oils or fatty foods exposed to excess heat. Protect your oils from excess exposure to heat or ambient air. Consume only raw fresh nuts to avoid damaged fats produced by excess heat. Store nuts and oils in the refrigerator if you don't plan to use them within a few days. Processed and rancid fats promote inflammation and lead to tissue damage and disease. Avoid consuming and cooking with vegetable oils derived from canola, sunflower, or safflower as they are easily damaged both on the shelf and through the cooking process.

Special Considerations for the FINE Food Plan

Detoxification Support

Food is the mainstay of robust detoxification support, transforming and clearing out toxins that we ingest or create internally. Because detoxification goes on 24/7, it is imperative that we feed it regularly, not just during popular seasonal "cleanses," occasional juicing, fasting, or other detox strategies. We need a daily supply of healthy fats, proteins, and nutrition from multi-colored plants in our diets to optimize detoxification. For a more detailed discussion, including specialized supplements to support detoxification, see my article, *A Detoxification Primer.*[23]

Gut Function and Microbiome Support

We must have healthy gut function to digest our food and assimilate the nutrients it provides for us. We must cultivate a healthy microbiome, the trillions of bacterial cells that live with us in our bodies. Fact is, we *are* our microbiome. Our cellular function and genetic expression are completely intertwined and interdependent. Imbalances in gut flora come about from antibiotic use, poor diets, and exposure to environmental toxins (including many medications).

---

[23] Karyn Shanks, MD. *A Detoxification Primer.* 2018. At https://karynshanksmd.com/2018/12/09/a-detoxification-primer/

The following are basic guidelines for optimizing gut and microbiome function with food.

- Eat in a relaxed, unhurried fashion, rather than on the run.

- Chew slowly and appreciate the flavors and textures of your food.

- Consider the use of digestive aids such as enzymes, betaine hydrochloric acid, digestive bitters, ox bile, or melatonin. Work with your trusted health practitioner to guide you in their use.

- Treat gut inflammation that can disturb the absorptive capacity of the small bowel.

- Remove food allergens and irritants from your diet through the FINE or GRIN food plans.

- Optimize gut nutrition. Consider the use of l-glutamine (major energy source for gut mucosal cells), in addition to optimal fat, protein, and micronutrients.

- Feed the microbiome: non-digestive sugars (or fiber) from plants will provide your gut bacteria with needed fuel. Probiotic supplements can be useful for microbiome recovery.

GRIN—THE GUT-IMMUNE RESTORATION INTENSIVE NUTRITION FOOD PLAN

The Gut-Immune Restoration Intensive Nutrition (GRIN) food plan is designed to help those with chronic inflammatory and autoimmune conditions take their healing to a deeper level.

The GRIN food plan is an extension of the FINE food plan, going a bit further by excluding additional food groups that are common irritants to the gut lining (thereby increasing intestinal permeability—see discussion below), as well as triggers for inflammation and toxicity.

The Perfect Storm of Autoimmunity

There are four core issues that contribute to the perfect storm of autoimmune disorders and their suffering:

1. Genetic susceptibility,

2. Impaired intestinal permeability and microbiome imbalances,

3. An immunological trigger (or multiple triggers), and

4. Energy deficit.

Genetic Susceptibility

The genetic susceptibility piece is hard to predict, poorly understood, and likely present in all of us to varying degrees and at different stages of our lives. We know through the science of epigenetics that genetic expression can be changed through the influence of an infinite array and interaction of environmental and lifestyle factors. This puts us all at risk for autoimmunity in the "right" circumstances.

Impaired Intestinal Permeability and Microbiome Imbalances

Impaired intestinal permeability is a product of our toxic world, medications, suboptimal lifestyle factors, and gut microbiome imbalances that injure and irritate the gut. We'll discuss this more in an upcoming section.

Immunological Triggers

Immunological triggers are common and hard to predict when they become significant enough to generate autoimmunity. Everything from emotional stress, trauma, to severe or persistent infections and allergies have been implicated in the genesis of autoimmune disorders.

HEAL KARYN SHANKS MD

Energy Deficit

Energy deficit is present in autoimmunity as both a potential trigger as well as a manifestation of the widespread damage to the brain-thyroid-adrenal-mitochondrial (BTAM) energy operating system caused by the inflammatory-autoimmune process. It is a feed-forward problem that accelerates and exacerbates the damage and suffering and must be addressed for healing to occur.

The Functions of the GRIN Optimal Energy Nutrition in Autoimmunity

- Repair and support of the BTAM energy operating system.

- Repair of the intestinal lining to restore normal permeability.

- Restoration of the gut microbiome.

- Downregulation of inflammation and autoimmune activity through shifts in genetic expression.

- Removal of common food-derived immunological triggers.

Who Needs to Follow the GRIN Food Plan?

This plan should be considered for anyone with persistent gut or inflammatory-autoimmune disorders who do not achieve optimal healing with the FINE Food Plan.

Chronic autoimmune disorders that respond beautifully to GRIN are:

- rheumatoid arthritis,

- lupus,

- Hashimoto's thyroiditis,

- celiac disease,

- multiple sclerosis,

- inflammatory bowel disease,

- ankylosing spondylitis,

- psoriasis, as well as others.

Autoimmunity Can Be Hidden

The GRIN food plan may also be appropriate for people with chronic disease or dysfunction without an obvious inflammatory component who fail to recover with less aggressive approaches.

Often inflammation is covert, without a readily recognized presentation, but may still be a factor. I see this in my practice frequently with people who have fatigue, chronic mood or cognitive dysfunction, or difficulty losing weight. They don't have sore joints or other signs of irritation in their bodies, but we know that inflammation can be a "hidden" player in these issues that respond well to anti-inflammatory approaches to healing.

How the GRIN Food Plan Works: Restoration of Normal Gut Permeability and Immune Function

A central theme to chronic inflammatory and autoimmune disorders is impairment of the gut lining that leads to increased gut permeability ("leaky gut"). This problem inevitably leads to an increase in immune cell responsiveness to food and gut microbes. It also leads to increased transfer of gut-derived or ingested toxins out of the gut and into the systemic circulation, engendering additional immune activation and inflammation.

A normal gut, some thirty feet long from mouth to anus, and the surface area of ten tennis courts, provides us with a very tightly controlled interface between the inside and outside worlds. As you can imagine, just as our skin is a crucial barrier for keeping the outside world out, the gut lining is designed to protect us from all potential threats, while at the same time selectively allowing in nutrients the body needs.

As vast as the gut interface is, the body must contribute more than seventy percent of its immune cells to stand guard along its borders. If the barrier is breached, there is an instantaneous response by immune cells. That response is complex and involves a direct attack to the offender as well as chemical signaling to attract other immune cells throughout the body, inviting them to participate in the protective response. This rapidly becomes a full-body process, amplifying protection as well as potentially spreading havoc from the gut to tissues throughout the body, as far away as the brain.

The gut lining can be damaged by many potential irritants and stressors. The susceptibility to injury varies from one person to the next.

Common Gut Lining Irritants and Stressors:

- anti-inflammatory drugs such as Ibuprofen, Aleve, aspirin, and steroids

- antibiotics

- alcohol

- acid-blocking drugs (like proton pump inhibitors and H2 blockers)

- heavy metals (from environmental contamination, contaminated food, dental mercury amalgams)

- infections (bacteria, parasites, fungi, viruses)

- food proteins

- excessive exercise

- excesses of stress

- persistent insomnia

- nutrient deficiencies and nutrient-poor diets

- microbiome imbalances

A leak of material that normally would not have access to the internal environment of the gut lining cells and intercellular spaces leads to a predictable immune response. This can escalate into a cascade of immune signaling and chemical action that rapidly becomes a systemic process, leading to the common symptoms of inflammation and global dysfunction, which for some can be catastrophic.

Current scientific thinking is that a key aspect of initiating and perpetuating chronic inflammatory and autoimmune disorders is activation of the immune response when the normal gut barrier is compromised.

Exposure of the immune cells that line the gut to ingested food components and toxins results in immune activation that begins and sustains the process.

To heal chronic inflammatory and autoimmune disorders we must heal the gut, restore normal gut permeability, and restore a healthier and more diverse microbiome.

Gut Healing Strategy to Reverse Autoimmunity

- Repair the gut lining through targeted nutrition and removal of toxins and irritants.

- Restore normal gut permeability.

- Restore normal digestion and absorption of nutrients.

- Restore a healthy microbiome.

- Decrease immune system responsiveness through food modulation and intensive targeted nutrition.

- Support energy production with energy nutrition.

This comprehensive gut healing effort, when combined with other approaches to reduce physical stress and restore immune balance, will lead to improvement and sustainable resolution of symptoms at a root cause level. The process involves many steps. Food is where we start.

GRIN Is Not Meant to Be a Lifelong Plan

The GRIN food plan is designed to heal your gut, remove the common triggers for inflammation, intensify nutrition, and reverse systemic symptoms related to gut-immune dysfunction and nutrient deficiencies.

GRIN is not meant to be a lifelong eating strategy.

The vast majority of people use this plan to heal, then are able to successfully reintroduce food groups into their diet without a recurrence of symptoms.

When working with clients one-on-one, I make personalized recommendations depending on how sick they've been and what their preferences are. It can be very helpful to have the support and experienced guidance from a Functional Medicine practitioner or functional nutrition professional. However, many people successfully navigate this journey on their own.

The Gut-Immune Restoration Intensive Nutrition (GRIN) Food Plan Details

The foundation for the GRIN food plan is FINE. We will be modifying that plan by excluding additional food groups that act as irritants to the gut and immune system.

Recall the Foods to Exclude in the FINE Food Plan:

- grains,

- animal milk products,

- processed foods,

- synthetic foods,

- preservatives,

- chemical additives,

- unhealthy meats,

- excesses of sugar, and

- unhealthy fats.

Recall the Foods to Include in the FINE Food Plan:

- Healthy meat choices, eggs, and fish;

- Non-starchy vegetables;

- Low sugar content fruit;

- Nuts and seeds;

- Bone broth;

- Spices, condiments, food supplements;

- Healthy fats;

- Beans and legumes;

- Teas;

- Fermented foods;

- Fluids;

- Smoothies;

- Appropriate nutritional supplements.

Additional Foods to Avoid on Your GRIN Food Plan

In addition, you will need to exclude the following foods and food groups: (But, remember, this food plan is not about deprivation—though it may feel like that right now—it's about substitution. Eat as much as you like, just of the good stuff.)

Eggs: Proteins contained in both the whites and yolks of eggs are common immunological triggers, commonly seen in the setting of impaired gut permeability. Avoid using eggs and all egg-containing products.

Beans and Legumes: This includes all beans, legumes (such as lentils and other dals), and dried peas. These contain abundant lectins on their surfaces, defense molecules that are known to trigger immune cells, resulting in inflammation and gut lining injury.

Nightshades: Nightshades are sources of alkaloids, plant defense molecules that can injure the gut lining. Avoid all white potatoes, tomatoes and tomato products, eggplants, sweet bell peppers (all colors), hot peppers, cayenne pepper, goji berries, paprika, pimentos, tomatillos and some curry powders (check ingredients!). Ashwagandha, an herb commonly contained in adrenal support formulas, is also a nightshade, so look at your supplements carefully.

Note: sweet potatoes and yams are fine to eat.

Nuts: Avoid all nuts and nut-derived oils. This includes almonds, walnuts, cashews, pecans, Brazil nuts, pine nuts, hazelnuts, and pistachios, along with all nut oils, flours, butters, and milks.

Alcohol: Alcohol is always a gut lining irritant and detoxification challenge in spite of evidence that it is health promoting when consumed in moderation. Avoid all alcohol in beverages as well as cooking during this initial intense phase of the food plan. Moderate alcohol consumption may be added later for many individuals.

Seeds: Seeds contain protease inhibitors, enzyme inhibitors which may contribute to maldigestion and gut lining irritation. In my experience, seeds seldom result in true food sensitivity, and can be eaten in quantities small enough that the protease inhibitors they contain should not create a problem. I generally allow them in the GRIN food plan, but recommend removing them if sufficient healing and symptomatic progress is not made otherwise.

Most Protein Supplements: The only commercially available protein supplements allowed during this intensive phase of your GRIN food plan are gelatin and collagen derived from grass-fed beef, hemp seed, and other seed-derived proteins (if allowed). I like the hydrolyzed collagen from Great Lakes. It is odorless, tasteless, and performs extremely well, dissolving completely in any liquid at any temperature. It can be added to veggie smoothies, soups, stews, bone broth, and all liquids you wish to consume.

GRIN Strategy and Reintroduction of Foods

As I said, GRIN is not meant to be a lifelong food plan. We want to put the fire of inflammation out and heal the gut. We want to build tolerance to foods and create resilience. And we want to create energy. Once healed, many people are able to put food groups back into their diet without recurrence of symptoms. Following are some simple guidelines for food reintroduction.

- Strictly adhere to the GRIN food plan guidelines for at least three months. Your body needs this time to remove immunological debris, heal damaged tissue, restore normal gut permeability, reestablish a healthy gut flora, and decrease the overall responsiveness to culprit foods.

- Keep a detailed daily log of food and symptoms.

- If your symptoms are not resolved by three months, keep going with the strict GRIN food plan and consult with a Functional Medicine professional.

- If your symptoms have resolved, choose the foods you would like to reintroduce first—do not plan to reintroduce gluten or animal milk products initially, or other foods you know for certain have caused you significant problems in the past.

- Start with just one food at a time:

- Have one healthy serving (one-half to one cup) of a pure form of the food you are reintroducing, for example one half cup of almonds or one cup of a nightshade vegetable.

- Do not eat more of your chosen foods (or other foods on your forbidden list) for three days as you carefully observe for symptoms that may be related to the introduced food.

- If you feel well, try it a second time, and this time eat one serving per day for a week, while not introducing any other foods you've been avoiding on GRIN. This will allow you to discover if your sensitivity to this food occurs gradually with repeated exposures. If all goes well, feel free to add this particular food back to your diet, but don't eat it every day (increases the risk of re-sensitizing to it). Instead plan to include it on a rotational basis every three to four days.

- If a food makes you feel unwell at any time during this process, stop eating it and strictly exclude it from your diet.

- Once you've finished exploring your first food, move on to a second in the same careful fashion. If you go too fast, you may end up with symptoms and not know which food caused them, necessitating going back to strict GRIN eating and starting this process over.

LAST THOUGHTS

Now, breathe. Go back to your strong center.

Feeling daunted? Bring in some help! Work with a nutrition specialist or physician trained in Functional Medicine (FM) and FM nutrition. This is big stuff and may involve big change—let a pro help you get knowledgeable, organized, and create a plan that fits you and your needs. Follow up with them as often as you need to create deep sustainable changes in the way you eat and live. And if the food changes leave you feeling deprived, learn to transform that powerful energy into something empowering—work with my deprivation exercise in appendix A.

Then, hold on to your seat! As you step into this arena of doing hard things, you're going to bump up against resistance. What's the source of this resistance? These are the stories—the *tenacious* stories—that get in the way of our healing. The stories of our power, our worth, our belonging, our fears (of change, and where change might lead us), and time. That's okay; it's all part of our human journey. Our journey of discovery of ourselves. Join me in the next chapter, DISCOVER—Realize Your Mind's Infinite Potential. We'll learn our minds are infinite. *We're* infinite. We can call our power back and claim our true life stories. We can heal.

Chapter Eight

DISCOVER

Realize Your Mind's Infinite Potential
(Claim Your True Life Stories)

Our minds are our greatest tools and advisors, but they are tricksters too.
Serving our highest intentions as well as survival. Who's the master?
Our higher, integrated selves know exactly who we are—whole, beautiful, strong.
While our survival-oriented brains jump into the past, and the future—making assumptions, weaving tales, fearing what has not yet come to pass. Creating anxiety to protect us from our worst-case scenarios.

Already whole, many of those stories disempower us—guilt, shame, hopelessness. They must be cast away.

Already beautiful, the stories of isolation or unworthiness are not ours—they never were. They must be rejected.

Already strong, the stories of helplessness and needing others to fix us make us forget our infinite potential and innate power to heal.

Yes, our minds are complex. Our minds can tell us conflicting stories. Our minds can hold us back.

But our minds are also infinite. We're infinite. We can call our power back. We can claim our true life stories. We can heal.

A STORY ABOUT *MY* LIFE STORY

When my oldest son was in high school, the students in his class were asked to pick the person they each most admired—their heroes—and write about them. He told me in his casual and offhanded way that he had chosen two people because he couldn't decide between them.

The first person he chose was Papa, his grandfather. This I so understood. My father-in-law was someone who overcame all odds to become a world famous neurosurgeon, was highly respected for his innovative work as well as for his kindness, commitment, and generosity. He was the tireless worker. The model scientist and clinician. Techniques he developed are in commonplace use today. And he was kind, patient, and loving. Although he has passed away, his students and patients still write to my mother-in-law every Christmas, remembering him and his effect on their lives. Papa was every bit the quiet hero.

But after my son told me he had picked Papa as one of his heroes, he said something else that floored me: his other hero was me.

And in his quiet, thoughtful, straightforward way, he explained why. "Of course, Mom (you dumb head!), look where you came from. You overcame so much in your life to achieve so much."

I was dumbstruck. I didn't just not know what to say, my brain simply couldn't recognize what he was talking about. I'm just *me*, Mom, not a hero. I do my best and am a good person—but a hero? Like Papa or the other amazing heroes his classmates chose? No way!

I can't overstate my shock and awe at my son's choice of me as one of his heroes. First, this was coming from a seventeen-year-old. He was already staking his claim as a young man, independent of his mom. There were times I wasn't sure if he even liked me (silliness on my part, but the whole teenage transition is hard). Second, not only had I never complained about my past struggles, I had purposefully protected both of my sons from parts of my story. I wanted my parents and my sons to forge their own bonds without my history getting in the way.

Where My Old Story Came From

Yes, I had challenges growing up. My son knew that I was on my own by the time I was seventeen, and that I left high school early because of bullying at the inner-city San Diego high school I went to. I was an undergraduate for eight years while I explored who I was and what I wanted to do. I panicked about whether I even belonged in college and didn't even know I was smart until I "accidentally" aced a science exam. Until then I was not at all confident about my ability to achieve and accomplish. I worked throughout college and paid my own way. I was so poor during those years, I'm not sure what I ate or how I clothed myself, but I managed.

I got an associate's degree in psychology from San Diego City College, then enrolled at San Diego State University as a nursing major. On the first day of my first class as a nursing student, the teacher said, "Nursing is not medicine." She was trying to say something positive about nursing, how it was more about human relationships than medicine, but I realized in that moment that I *wanted* to be in medicine. Being a doctor wasn't anything I had ever dreamed of or imagined I could do. But then, I started to dream. And when I applied to medical school at the University of Chicago, I got in. That in itself was a miracle to me, but was further miraculous because it was where I met my future husband and my boys' father.

Since then my proudest accomplishment has been creating a safe, loving, and nurturing home for my family. But I never for a moment thought of myself as a hero. That wasn't my story.

But as well as I knew my story, as certain as I was of its details, my son saw something different.

A Young Boy Sees Me Through a Fresh Lens

He knew there was a lot of challenge and stress for me growing up. He watched me build my own medical practice. As a young boy he hung out at the office after school while I worked and heard all about how I worried and researched and went to bat for my patients who had chronic complex illnesses. He lived and grew and thrived within the embrace of my greatest legacy, our family, our home, and what we all created together.

From a place of unconditional love, stability, and calm, my son had observed all that went on around him. To my surprise, he saw me—*really saw me*—and many of the details of my life. And his conclusion was that I was a hero.

My Son Taught Me a New Life Story

My son's clarity and love and admiration blew my mind right open. He made me realize that there was an entirely different way to understand my life, one that he could see and that I had failed to. This idea catapulted me out of my old life story.

As we'll talk about in this chapter, we all have our life stories. It's how we see, understand, and relate to all that's happening to us. It's the framework through which we view all the various aspects of our lives—bodies, minds, and spirits.

My life story—the one I claimed for myself—had been one of shame and abandonment. It was a story of unworthiness and working hard to compensate. But through my son's clarity and love and admiration, he delivered a message in a way that cut through all my layers of hardwired dogmatic self-judgment to change how I felt.

Through him, I learned that my story is a story of freedom. My story is a story of courage. My story is a story of a scrappy girl finding her way early in life and how that taught her essential skills she would not have otherwise learned. That forced her to decide for *herself* what was right instead of being tethered to the conventional norms of society or those of her family.

Seeing My Life Through the Lens of Love

I saw that every experience, every bit of that past that I had previously believed had held me back, had actually taught me important lessons, cultivated strength in me, and made me who I am today. It was Life School, and it prepared me to do what I'm doing today.

Thanks to my son, I was able to take my old story and transform it into one that was more ennobling, that looked at my past through the lens of love. But I've since learned it doesn't have to take a spectacular revelation like I had to figure these things out. We just have to understand that everything we believe about ourselves and our lives *are* stories— stories that may not contain all the facts. How truthful are they *really*? How well do they serve our highest good?

Healing My Story Meant There Was Work to Do

To fully embrace my new story, there was much work to do. There was a lot of muck to clear out: I had to let go of blame, accept responsibility for who I was, and claim the freedom and power that I had even back then. To realize that *nothing anyone did to me was personal*. It was not about me. Not any of it.

Healing

I finally understood that *I* get to decide who I am and what I'm worth. I had courage and I rose up out of difficult times. And I'm pretty cool. Pretty damned cool. Through the clear eyes of my precious son, through the eyes of love, I see myself as a hero. And it is through that lens of love that I've come to choose to see myself and to see others and life itself.

OUR MINDS WERE DESIGNED FOR STORYTELLING

Stories are powerful things. They're how we see, understand, and relate to all that's happening to us. They're the framework through which we view all aspects of our lives—our minds, emotions, bodies, and spirits.

These stories of ours can represent our power—they can strengthen, fortify, and nourish our healing journey. But our stories can also stop us soundly in our tracks.

Stories Contain Our Wisdom

In times before writing, stories were how people passed down knowledge, wisdom, and aspirations. Even now, we listen to stories at the feet of our parents and remember them to tell our children. We read and listen as we share common stories across time and across culture. Stories are the very breath of our humanity and our spirit.

Stories Keep Us Alive

As we've developed as a species, stories have also kept us alive. Is the rustling in the grass next to us a tiger or just the wind? Is the withering of the leaves just the first signs of fall or a failure of the harvest? Being able to understand what is happening now and remembering it in exquisite detail in the future has great survival value.

We're Wired for Stories

When you consider how useful stories have been to our species, it's not hard to see that we are wired to create them. They're in our DNA. They're how our brains evolved to help us work and succeed. Our prefrontal cortex, the large front part of our brains, distinguishes us as humans, and is designed for storytelling. We call this our intellect. It endows us with the ability to pull together all the available data from our lives and rapidly arrive at an understanding about what's going on, followed by a plan and action.

"The" Truth is Really "Our" Truth

Stories and their lessons can save us in times of danger. Most of the time, however, we aren't in any *real* danger. But we still make rapid, unconscious assessments about what's going on that serve as the foundation for our beliefs and understanding. We do this all the time. Many of our assessments are laser sharp and spot on. But jumping to conclusions can be wildly problematic under the more ordinary circumstances of our lives.

We often forget that our stories reflect our own uniquely biased interpretations of the facts rather than the facts themselves. Our stories represent only a singular view (our own) of what's happening. We're all familiar with the well-known observation that groups of people looking at the very same set of circumstances (a crime, for instance), tell vastly different accounts of what happened. The details of their stories were determined by the unique lenses through which they saw the facts.

We draw conclusions about our subjective understanding of what the facts mean. We create stories, calling them "understanding," or "the truth," or "how it is." But there is danger in holding on too tightly to what we think we know for sure.

We are often lured into believing that our stories *are* the facts themselves. But, really, our stories are assumptions *about* the facts—assumptions that may be incomplete, or not at all true. And in limiting ourselves to these assumptions, we lock in the story, not leaving room for something better to emerge.

Our Life Stories Are Not Fixed

When I had the chance to see my own life through a new lens and tell myself a new story—a positive and beautiful and shiny story—everything changed. I see the old things differently. I relate the elements with love, not judgment. And new things that are bright get even shinier as I add them to my brilliant story.

Understand that this is not a choice to see things through rose-colored glasses. It's a conscious choice to reframe the facts as we know them and to allow that we don't have *all* the facts. It's the perspective shift of a mature mind.

We Can Unleash Our Potential

We are never trapped by our stories. We do not have to be limited, defined, or maligned by our stories. While we are powerfully influenced by them, *we* are not our beliefs or our stories. They are *constructs* of our brains. We create them, but they are not *us*.

And this is our ultimate point of control over our lives to claim our energy, healing, and potential.

Stories on the Brain: Neural Networks and Neuroplasticity

Our stories have a biology. In the body we call stories *neural networks*—brain pathways that integrate all our experiences, learning, and beliefs. These pathways are comprised of specialized nerve cells and the connections between those cells. They converge to create meaning (stories) and strengthen function in response to the incoming "data" of our lives.

Our brains and their neural networks change from moment to moment. The biological energy behind this change is called *neuroplasticity*. This process operates constantly to shape structure and function. It is influenced by our thoughts, memories, intentions, actions, and condition of our health.

Given the right circumstances (say, a healthy body, and loving, positive, hopeful outlook), neuroplasticity is the promise of how our brains can change to serve and support our best lives.

Learning to Walk: Neuroplasticity and Locomotion

A universal example of neuroplasticity is how we learn to walk by ourselves as small children, with no prior experience. No one really teaches us to walk. We yearn for the motion that will transport us toward what we are curious about. We struggle and experiment and fail, but we don't give up. Our practice leads to the development of the neural networks of locomotion. Our brains change as the circuitry for strength, balance, coordination, and muscle memory grows and expands. We gradually, miraculously, master this complex skill. The energy of neuroplasticity lays down the neural networks to support the growth and precision of our new skill.

We Build Stories the Same Way

We create and guide the development of stories in the same way that we learn a physical skill, like walking. Through the genius of neuroplasticity, what we learn, remember, imagine, decide, and do, all converge to create and strengthen our stories. Like walking, with enough practice, our stories become our reality.

If our tendency is to ruminate about all the bad things that have happened to us, we're practicing a negative way of being. We strengthen the neural networks that perceive our life stories through a negative lens (self-condemnation, disempowerment, being a victim, for example). Our brains will operate according to these "facts." We will persist in seeing our lives this way ("the way it is"), and all new experiences will be seen through this lens, reinforcing the old stories and limiting our ability to change.

Neuroplasticity: Our Hope to Succeed at Change

Neuroplasticity is also what gives us the ability to change our stories—not the facts, but our stories about those facts. If we practice perceiving our life stories through a positive lens (brave, scrappy, hopeful), our brains enter this data into our neural networks, and we see the world more brightly. We add new experiences to our stories that reinforce the positive, and we realize there are no limits to what we can do.

In other words, we can consciously *choose* to create new, more positive life stories—by harnessing the energy of neuroplasticity through our intentions and actions. The new neural networks of our creation will compete for space in our brains, growing and strengthening as we practice.

The take-home? Our brains and our bodies *quite literally* change as a direct result of our thoughts, intentions, and actions. Our potential function evolves by how we practice. We can apply this power to any aspect of our lives we want to change. By actively choosing and defining our stories and the lens through which we choose to see the world, we can change our physical being.

Passively Living Our Stories Invites Chaos and Fear

Our brains are an organization much like a business. In the business world it's said that all organizations have a "culture." A culture is the way things are done, the written or *unwritten* rules that everyone knows.

Sometimes a culture is consciously developed by the organization, but even if an organization doesn't actively work to build a specific, desired culture, one will still exist. It will be random, undefined, unclear, and may very well work *against* the organization's goals.

Stories are just like that. We *all* have stories—at every moment, about *everything*. They may serve us well or they may not.

We can reflect on our lives and consciously develop and define our stories, or we can passively accept what comes. Although it may seem easier, our brains are designed to be defensive, to keep us from harm, to be afraid. Fear is the path of least resistance and the way our brains were designed to keep us alive.

So, the default stories our brains keep coming back to will be fearful. This phenomenon is widely known in psychology as our brain's innate "negativity bias."

BIG STORIES THAT STAND IN THE WAY OF OUR HEALING

Okay, so we know that we have the power to heal by changing our stories. We have the science that explains the biology of it. We have the life experiences to lay the foundation of our stories. All the information we need is right here at our fingertips to lead us on a journey of profound healing and energy restoration. So, why don't we just do it? What stands in our way?

Remember these stories from our previous chapters?

I can't.

I don't have time.

Who am I to... ?

These are the preambles we use to explain how we've become stuck in the face of our common and powerful life stories. These are the stories that stomp on our lives and sap our souls. Here's what they sound like, in their various forms, as my clients say them out loud in my consultation room:

Powerful Stories of Being Stuck

- "There is nothing more that can be done for me." (Says who? You're the expert on you!)

- "I am a diabetic." "I am depressed." "This is who I am." (Really? I thought you were an artist named Sarah, not a diagnosis.)

- "My doctor knows best." (Does she? Who says? I'll bet she makes mistakes too.)

- "My symptoms are all in my head." (So is your insightful and incredibly intelligent brain! What's it telling you about your symptoms?)

- "I'm just like my mother (or father)—this is my destiny." (Epigenetics, anyone? Your genes are not your destiny!)

- "I am trapped." (No, hon, you've just lost the creativity to find a way to move on. Let's get that creativity back as a first step.)

- "I am alone." (Not anymore! There's a whole bunch of us working through this and we're happy to welcome you along.)

- "I can't change." (You already have. You decided to read this! Congratulations on your first steps.)

- "My diagnosis is..." (Your diagnosis is just a name, perhaps just a symptom. Tell me about you.)

These are all very real stories I've been told. Are any of them familiar to you?

They are beliefs and assumptions that are held as *the truth*, but are not based on all the facts, or any facts at all. They're stories based on judgments and fears that are learned, latched onto, and become obstacles to positive change and healing. We adopt them unconsciously from our experiences, perceptions, and the world around us. They may accurately reflect how we *feel* or what we truly believe, but they are not *the truth*. They can all be changed.

Five Life Stories that Slam the Brakes on Healing

To help us think about how to get past some of the major roadblocks to healing, I want to focus on five different stories that often get us stuck. It is important to remember that each of these stories, while often fearful products of our cautious primal brains, can also become stories of strength and potential for growth:

- The story of our power.

- The story of our worth.

- The story of how we belong.

- The story of our fear about uncertainty and change.

- The story of not having enough time.

These are the stories of our lives that must be reckoned with to see ourselves as we are, filled to the brim with potential. These are the stories that must be transformed for Big Energy and healing to become ours.

The Story of Our Power

"I am the expert on me."

We have lost the idea that we can heal ourselves. We turn to others who know more than we do, who have more experience than we do, who do this "for a living." But none of them knows us better than we know ourselves. None of them has more experience in being us than we do.

Our healthcare professionals are certainly skilled and valued. I honor them all. But, none of them are an expert on *me*. They practice for the masses. They have to. And if in times of acute crisis, I need their help, I turn to them gratefully.

But the world is changing. As we've established, most of our illnesses are now chronic. The very real need for fast short-term treatments that drove the development of modern acute-care medicine through the last century is no longer what most of us need. But we still turn to the principles and players of acute care every day. We turn to the experts. We look for the single cure (like the abnormal thyroid test I longed for). But if we don't find it, we're out of luck. Who do we turn to then? Who's the expert?

In the past, before the voices of those many experts drowned out our own, we *knew* who to turn to—*ourselves*. We *knew* what we needed and *knew* how to heal. Our own inner wisdom guided us through all but the most acute and catastrophic of illnesses.

None of us are immune to our culture, to the stories that tell us "how things are." But in the modern world, many of the most destructive stories lead us to believe that forces beyond ourselves and out of our control are in charge of our health and healing.

As a physician with nearly three decades of experience, working with clients with complex chronic illnesses (often referred from the universities who don't know what to do with these folks), I don't believe any of these myths. Not only are they untrue, they sit squarely in the way of healing.

Only by claiming our power and agency over our own lives can we capture the healing and energy recovery we seek.

The Story of Our Worth

"I deserve and must have my reverent attention and care."

These common stories of judgment, blame, and toxic shame slam the door on our healing every time:

- Who am I to make my needs a top priority?

- Who am I to ask for help?

- My illness makes me less valuable to my family, friends, and tribe.

We learn these disempowering stories from our tribes and soak them up from our culture. We adopt them as our own. But they're not ours. And they're *never* true. Not ever. We're *born* worthy.

Inherently complete, lovable, and whole, just as we are. Not needing to be "fixed." Not needing permission from someone else to be who we are.

Our inherent worth is right here inside us, having just gotten lost and fallen out of sight. Buried beneath fatigue and overwhelm or drowned out by the noise of our stories. Stories of unworthiness. Stories we've practiced, and through our practice, strengthened. Stories engendering neural networks of shame and blame, burying the essential truth that we are whole and holy. As we are.

Permission Slip: Permission to Be Your Whole True Self

We begin here: with permission. Permission to acknowledge our worthiness and wholeness. Permission to unwind the mind pathways of shame and strengthen those of love and self-acceptance. Write yourself this permission slip (or your own version) and read it out loud when you're done. I have many such permission slips written on sticky notes that I carry around with me.

Dear [your name here],

I give you my full permission to be your whole, true, authentic self—just as you are, right now. Already whole. Already lovable. Already beautiful. Already complete. Welcome home. You belong here. Safe. No guilt. No shame. Already enough. Only love.

The Story of How We Belong

"I stand tall and strong and courageous on my personal healing journey."

We're genetically wired to belong to our families, tribes, and communities. Strong communal ties kept our ancestors alive when being left behind or ostracized meant certain death. This is still true today for many people living in inner cities, refugee camps, and abusive family relationships, places where survival is tested every day. And protecting our children within the safety of our tribes will always be crucial.

However, for most of us, the reality of our modern world is that our survival is not so fragile. Whether we live on the edge or in more comfortable surroundings, our evolutionary experience has shaped the development of our brains so feeling safe and secure is strongly tied to the bonds of our births, allegiances, shared beliefs, and ways of living.

Beyond survival, we find comfort belonging to the friends who share pizza and beer together on Friday nights. We gain strength belonging to the work community who collaborate, share stories by the water cooler, and burn the midnight oil together. We grow along with our badassed comrades pounding it out at the gym. We cherish belonging to the families who love one another through food or seal their ties through shared beliefs and behaviors. It feels good. It feels comfortable. It feels safe.

Our deepest inner beingness thrives through these connections.

We Bravely Take a Stand for Our Own Healing

But this healing life we've chosen asks us to make new choices.

We *must* change the things that need to be changed.

We may choose not to eat pizza or drink beer. We may choose to create a more balanced life of work and play and self-care. We may make choices that go against the grain of our pack.

But to claim healthier choices in the face of what our friends, co-workers, and family are doing can seem radical, challenging those relationships, inspiring scrutiny and criticism, breaking seemingly vital bonds.

However good and imperative our choices may be, we may feel lonely and scared as we bravely take a stand for our own healing.

To Whom Do We Belong?

This is one of the tests of our healing life: to whom do we belong?

How do we survive when our path to healing challenges us to stand apart from the crowd? How do we quiet their voices so we can hear our own? How do we make choices and take actions that are best for us but make us stand out or leave us behind?

Beyond the choices we make and the outcomes we expect, we still wonder:

- What happens when we become well?

- How does our vibrant new energy, happiness, or ideal body weight effect our relationships?

- Will our friends and family support us and cheer us on?

- Will we get backlash from their misplaced jealousy, anger, or their own feelings of abandonment?

Our Healing Story: We are Strong and Brave

But while these feelings are normal, they're not our whole story: *we are also strong and brave.* And as we've discussed throughout this book, our deepest inner beingness also requires:

- Our strong singular presence.

- Our own mind.

- Our self-focused heart.

- Our strong center.

The end to our suffering means courageously embracing our true authentic selves. To live this healing life we've chosen, we're called to *belong to ourselves*. We must use that strong center we've worked so hard to find, connect to, and nourish. We must shine a bright light on our lives and use our own minds and hearts to decide what's best for our healing.

Brave souls called to belong to themselves soon learn:

- Loneliness is temporary and not fatal.

- The backlash of others is not personal.

- Our anxiety is just energy.

- The rewards are eternal.

Remember what happens when we care for ourselves first?

Yes, we're stronger, wiser, more resilient, and vibrant. We live and lead through the radiance of our healing lives. We pave the road for others.

We Share This Healing Path with Many Others

And we soon realize there's a reward we may not have expected: we're surrounded by companions living their own healing lives. We take this journey both alone and with the strength, nourishment, and companionship of others. While we may let go of those who no longer support us, we're joined by new travelers in this healing life. This can be hard, but it's the only true life. It's the only life in which we can claim the healing and potential that are ours.

Exercise: Expedition to the Terrain of our True Authentic Selves

What if you could practice the call to belong to yourself? To prepare for those times when the way is unclear or when the road gets treacherous? To stand up to the scrutiny of your critics?

We've practiced this before: we slip into our strong center. This is the strong center we know well, that we've already claimed as our own. It's the space of belonging to ourselves. Everything we've learned to do to support it makes us strong and brave in the face of life's challenges.

Let's drop into our strong center now. Place your hands over your midsection. Take a few slow deep breaths into your core. Ah, yes, this is me. This is us. This is our strength.

Say this: I can stand alone here. I can weather any storm, any journey, any challenge from this place of strength. In choosing to be here, I belong. I belong to myself. I belong to my tribe of companions on this healing journey. I choose what's best for me without distraction or interference. I trust my strength and wisdom to fortify me as I become more and more my whole, true, authentic self. As I steadily rise into my true potential, I trust my light, which I radiate all around me. This is the light that allows my travel companions to find me, and for me to see them. In being true to myself—belonging to myself—I am never truly alone.

The Story of Our Fear about Uncertainty and Change

"My potential for growth, healing, and successful change are infinite."

All efforts to heal require change, and that means an unknown outcome. Always.

We see our problem—we're not where we want to be yet. We know what we *aspire* to (energy recovery, getting our lives back). We know *what* we want to change (starting with our life stories). We know there is a roadmap (the Nine Domains of Healing) that will guide us. And we know there is a community that will be with us to support us and share our journey. We know that others (many others) have succeeded at doing this.

Change is Scary

But change still scares us.

It's been said that all change begets mourning. Change is a loss. We have to give something up, abandon our old familiar ways, whether they serve us well or not. No matter how bad something is, it's ours, it's comfortable, it's the way things have been. We know it. We can count on it. We've built our life around it. We know how to survive with it. And maybe all our energy has gone into surviving by keeping things the same.

To change, we are challenged to learn something new. To change, we may be called upon to do something hard. To change, we must step up to an unknown outcome—we might fail.

Change is Our Only Sources of Untapped Potential

In his book *The Discoverers*, Daniel Boorstein writes a different story about change: "The most promising words ever written on the maps of human knowledge are terra incognita, unknown territory."

What he's saying is that moving into the unknown is the only thing that releases us, giving us the promise of untapped potential. It's our freedom. It's how we change our story to find our energy and healing.

It's important to remember that change is not only what we can do now, it's what we've been doing since the day we were born. Just as healing and love are parts of us, so too is succeeding at change. When you learned to walk—wow, what a change. What amazing new potential!

Our fear-of-change stories often operate on a subconscious level, making them more destructive because we often aren't aware that they're sabotaging our efforts to create positive change. But if we follow the fear to that story, if we can unpack it and see it for what it is—the product of our imagination and assumptions—we open up the opportunity to create a better story. A story that supports our healing.

What Our Fear-of-Change Stories Look Like

Think about some ways in which fear can get in the way of healing. Think of some ways fear might make you question the decision to focus on your health.

- Here are some fear-of-change stories I've heard from my clients:

- What will be required of me if I feel really good? Will I have to go back to that job I hate?

- How will feeling well change my relationships? Will my loved ones still take care of me? Will they still love me?

- How will succeeding at feeling well change me? I'm afraid of who I will become.

- If I am strong and healthy, will others feel jealous of me? Will I still belong?

- If I am strong and healthy, I will be amazing and powerful. That scares me.

Are you squirming yet? These commonly held unconscious stories can be the most difficult because they expose areas of our lives where we feel profoundly vulnerable. At the root of these stories are assumptions about our physical and emotional safety and survival. About our place within our tribes, our families. About our worth and lovability. About our personal power and creativity.

All Our Fearful Stories Can Be Rewritten:

- What will be required of me if I feel really good? What new exciting opportunities will show up that I haven't even thought of yet?

- How will feeling well change my relationships? How much richer will they be when I have this extra energy to put into them?

- How will succeeding at feeling well change me? When I build on this success, what other tasks can I take on and succeed at?

- If I am strong and healthy, I can be a role model for those I love.

- If I am strong and healthy, I will be amazing and powerful. That excites me.

Our minds and brains are amazing in the ways they innately step in to protect us from danger and deep suffering. However, to heal, we must transform our fearful stories with gentle self-awareness and loving softening. The smallest shifts can open the doors to hope, love, and infinite potential.

The Story of Not Having Enough Time

"I always have time for what I care about."

In chapter two, we talked about the distractions that sap our time, leading us to the false conclusion that we don't have enough of it. We discussed simple ways to create more time by letting go of the barrage of distractions and disruptions we often allow into our lives.

We also use "having no time" as an excuse for not taking the steps we need to create change. What's with that?

It all ties back to what we've just discussed—disempowerment, unworthiness, belonging, and fear of uncertainty. "I have no time" is often our euphemism for "I'm scared."

No more. We can't use that excuse anymore. We may consciously choose to put off the change we need. It may be all too much right now. Often times those baby steps are best. But no way are we going to lie to ourselves. We now know those untrue stories dismantle our power and our futures. To heal, we must become truth warriors. No excuses. No lies.

And beware of pretending *not* to suffer by numbing ourselves into oblivion—this saps *all* our time.

To make conscious choices about our healing, we must stand strong in our centers—whole, true, authentic, worthy. In this way we create time. We *always* have time, and we revere and amplify it by ditching distractions and excuses.

WE CAN CHANGE OUR BIG STORIES

Yes, You're Wired for Better Stories

The physiological reality is that, while our brains are wired to *resist* change to avoid uncertain and potentially dangerous circumstances, we are also wired to *succeed* at change. We all possess the deep potential of neuroplasticity—the engine of change that we've been discussing. Harnessing this potential requires only our imaginations, intentions, and actions.

Whatever we *conceive* of to change (imagination), whatever we *decide* to change (intention), and whatever we *practice* (action), *will* become manifest in our lives. This is certain.

Our brains know how to change. *We* know how to change. In one way or another we've been doing it every moment of our entire lives (change is the only certainty in life).

But, like our stories, change can be passively accepted or actively guided. One way can work *for* us, one against.

Although you may not see it yet, you're built for this work. You are a change warrior. You have powerful internal tools and resources to claim this for yourself.

Lay the Groundwork for Healing Your Stories

Remember when we learned what to pack and what to leave behind for our healing journey? The same is true for healing our stories. We've got to have the gear that strengthens us. And we've got to leave behind the baggage that slows us down.

Claim Your Inner Wisdom and Guidance

Yes, we *all* have inner wisdom, but many of us don't trust it or we don't stop to listen to it in the midst of our complicated, noisy lives. You must create time, space, and quiet to listen into your inner wisdom. It takes courage to step up to the truth and inner knowing of your wise center. It may set you apart from the other voices in your head and in your life.

Cultivate Optimism, Hope, and Faith

Humans may be wired for assuming the worst-case scenario when confronted with a challenging or stressful situation. But, really, these life-threatening situations are few and far between. Most of our lives are spent in risk-free moments. And in those many moments, whether we are aware of it or not, we also believe in a better future. This is what allows us to plan, to move forward, to get up in the morning. We always assume a better day is coming.

Having hope is vital for the healing process. Hope is the opening in our thinking that something better is possible, that healing is possible. We may not see it or know what it is, but we believe in the possibilities.

However, as adults, we know that our intentions seldom match the outcomes precisely.

So, while we use hope to bolster our potential—to prepare and energize us for the work to come—we need something else, something larger than we are.

I'm talking about hope's wiser sister: faith.

Hope is hard work. Faith, on the other hand, allows us to rest by assuring us that no matter what the outcome, we've done our very best. Faith softens us and lends us courage to forgive our disappointments and let go of our unrealized expectations. Faith is our maturity to receive the grace, the mercy, and all the stuff of life that comes as a result of—and in spite of—our best efforts.

Be Courageous

Whether we remember it or not, every single one of us has stepped up to a challenge. We've been courageous, and we can be so again. We may have fallen or failed. But we did our best even when we were scared or uncertain.

Be Curious

Curiosity is our birthright. Children are the greatest explorers of all time. We can't stop them! They take bold steps into terra incognita very day, sometimes giggling, sometimes falling down and giving a quick cry, but *always* getting back up. We must reclaim that potential for ourselves.

Curiosity moves us forward and is an absolute part of who we are. Admittedly, some adults don't *feel* curious anymore. But it's not because they've lost it. It's because it's been buried. It's really, truly in there. Rediscovering curiosity will be one of the joys of our work together. Whether you feel it there or not, be absolutely certain that it's there, and will emerge to lead you toward creative ideas and solutions.

Draw on Past Successes

Anything we do today will build on what we've done before. To develop and empower the amazing changes coming into your life, you will be building on all the successful changes you've managed before.

There may be a few failures along the way as well. That's fine! Welcome to being completely and utterly human. But please recognize that these "failures" are also rich experiences to draw insight from. One way to look at failure is as a huge punctuation mark where you must pause to see the opportunity or the better way. Learning what *doesn't* work is as valuable as learning what *does* work. In this way, life is all one big experiment (without the judgment). We'll work more deeply with failure in our final chapter.

Be Humble and Truthful

The scary, but necessary, part of self-discovery is seeing the parts of us that we don't like or that make us feel vulnerable. It's hard. But not nearly as hard as getting to the end of our lives and finding that we failed to step into our power and the deeper levels of our healing and happiness because we chickened out. We have to let go of our pride and always tell ourselves the truth. We must step into our adult minds. Those parts of us that we feel the most vulnerable about are often our greatest assets—our love, tenderness, compassion—our feelings. We need to know these things. The world needs them.

Claim Responsibility

To believe that I was a hero, as told to me through my son's perspective, I not only had to reckon with my assumptions about the events of my life being personal, I also had to claim personal responsibility for everything that happened to me and all of the choices I subsequently made. I had to claim this power for myself. I was half-assed about this for years, continuing to hustle for my sense of worth through blame, excuses, and numbing my pain in relentless hard work. It wasn't until I established a daily writing and meditation practice—creating the space for me to feel and breathe and find my center— that I was able to fully claim my power.

We must let go of the idea that through blame and excuses we complete our life story. That if we met misfortune, there must be someone to blame. This is almost never the case. I'm not talking about senseless acts of violence or damaging recklessness. I'm talking about all the rest of the events of our lives, the disappointments that we cling to by tethering ourselves to the past events and the people in them through blame. Or the excuses we carry with us to explain why we can't make the changes that will lead to healing.

Blame and excuses are our way of not having to step into our power. Blame and excuses are how we let go of personal responsibility for our lives. Blame and excuses suck our energy. They crush us. We must let them go right now.

Commit

You know this one, because you've said "yes," many times by now!

The most reliable and universal predictor of success that I observe in my clients is their willingness and ability to commit to their healing and to themselves. The *decision* to change ignites all healing.

This is also what *sustains* our healing: commitment is the decision to see our healing through, all the way to the very end. Starting is the easy part. Our decision to change—to heal—must be made every day.

Trust That Healing Is Your Innate Potential

We've talked about this before too. Healing is our innate, unstoppable potential, and a primary urge of nature. All things heal. And this healing that is our birthright can be passively accepted or actively directed. But we're also called to understand that healing is not always curing—while we may reach our heretofore unimagined potential through our reverent self-care, we may still have scars, suffering, and vulnerabilities that will require our lifelong care.

Practice

What you *do* is your story.

If you don't like your current story—change it. Create the vision, make the decision, then do it.

This is your power. How your simple decision, ignited by action, changes your stories, changes your mind, changes your neural networks, creates your new life.

The *real* story will always be in *the story you live*. Now. I love the old expression, "We make the road by walking." Gotta start walking.

IS THERE A TENACIOUS STORY STANDING IN YOUR WAY?

How do we know what's stalled our healing? How do we know if our "reality" is a story that's not supporting us? What do we look out for? This is not easy. Our minds can be tricky.

Remember all the dangerous stories that we've discussed in this chapter. For some of us, getting unstuck is a matter of finding the resources and support that we need but haven't had thus far. New information, education, or ideas may be just what we need to jumpstart a new phase to our healing. We may revitalize a stuck healing journey through a new perspective or direction of a new resource, mentor, or consultant. We can add new members to our team or call in the support of family and friends to help us.

But what if we're stuck with a tenacious story and can't see it?

Clues There May Be a Tenacious Story Standing in the Way of Your Healing:

- You know precisely how to solve your problem but just can't get it done. *Story*.

- You feel stuck. *"I'm stuck" is always a story*.

- You're afraid to commit to change you know you need. *Fear is a story*.

- You feel unlovable, undeserving, guilty, hopeless, or shameful. *Always a story!*

- You worry your loved ones won't support your healing. *Big assumptions. Big story.*

- You've done it all but are still suffering. *This is the most tenacious story of all. This is a story of fatigue, of suffering, of not seeing the way forward. I know you've worked hard, and it's been a long road, but I promise you haven't done it all. There is always a path forward. There's always space for change, for compassion and love, for progress.*

Beware of the Diagnosis—Certainty Is Always a Story

Uncertainty is scary.

But guess what? *Certainty*, while strangely comforting, is an even bigger problem.

Like the medical diagnosis, often declared with an air of certainty, naming something is a story, and can stop all inquiry and progress.

A diagnosis—or lack thereof—as proclaimed by your doctor (or other authoritative resource) can distract from the critical journey of understanding yourself and discovering the true meaning of your symptoms and problems as unique and distinct from everyone else's.

The diagnosis is a label—*a story*—that you are given as a way to explain your illness. Its purpose is to clarify the problem and provide direction for finding solutions. The diagnosis can provide a sense of comfort and certainty that your illness is "this thing," for which there is a predetermined path for resolution.

Sometimes this is exactly what happens: the clarity of the diagnosis leads directly to an effective treatment plan.

But by virtue of naming anything, the suggestion is that the problem is well defined, simple, and fully knowable. Except humans are complex.

The Diagnosis Oversimplifies the Problem

The diagnosis often oversimplifies the problem, failing to recognize the deeper causes. It gives us the illusion that we understand something that may actually defy full understanding. Or that changes. Or that has not been fully illuminated.

If the diagnosis were a hypothesis and not the final declaration of what is true, then it would be more helpful. It would serve as a guidepost, a useful roadmap in the process of discovery: "Here is what the data as we know it suggests." "Here is the hypothesis at this time about what is going on." "Let's investigate that."

The diagnosis should declare what we know so far, provide suggestions for a sense of direction, and *temporarily* simplify the problem so we can tend to one thing at a time (but not forget to come back to the big picture).

Pretending we are certain about something too complex to understand completely is harmful. It provides comfort but limits progress. It simplifies but restricts possibilities. It defines but doesn't tell the whole truth.

The Lack of Diagnosis is Also a Story

Likewise, the lack of diagnosis is a story that can get in the way of healing. When our doctors don't know what's wrong with us, or if we don't fit neatly into an existing diagnostic category, we're often told there is nothing wrong, or there is nothing more that can be done, or, still worse, our problems are all in our heads.

To Heal, Insist on the Truth of Uncertainty

For healing, rather than certainty, we need the truth of uncertainty (the truth that there is very little we know for sure) to inspire curiosity and inquiry. Only this truth can lead us to the deep, sustainable solutions we seek.

STORY MINING

Let's take a close look at those tenacious stories that have you stuck and mine them for the nuggets of gold and wisdom that will help you change and heal. We've got power tools to help you and a safe step-by-step strategy to guide you all the way through.

Power Tools for Story Mining

Take these tools with you everywhere. Use them to scrutinize everything you believe as you evaluate why you are stuck, scared, or unable to move forward with your healing. These are perspective changers. They don't change the facts, but they allow you to see the facts of your life through different lenses. These are lenses that let you cut through the muck, the bullshit, and the lies that cling to your truth—your *real* truth, the truth that will set you free.

- The lens of love.

- Life School point of view (POV).

The Lens of Love

When we understand our stories through a more positive and ennobling lens, everything changes. Love changes everything. It changes our brains, changes our genetic expression, and it changes our stories through a foundational perspective shift, not by conjuring new facts. Through the power of neuroplasticity to change our neural networks, love changes our futures and opens up possibilities for growth and healing that are impossible in its absence.

Love is broad and unlimited. Love of our families. Love of nature. Love of the littlest things in a day. Most importantly, love of ourselves. We are worthy and deserve a loving life story. There is nothing more you need—not the approval of someone else, not the permission of someone else, not someone else's story about us.

Each of us, in this moment, is filled with love. It's who we are. It's the lens we'll use to retell our stories—the lens we'll use to heal.

As we've discussed before, the reality is that many of us may be struggling or suffering in life and not able to *feel* love at this particular moment. Exhaustion and suffering make it hard to feel much of anything. But we can still practice. We can take small steps to build the neural networks of love. We can shift the overwhelmed, pessimistic thoughts to more hopeful ones.

The lens of love is what I learned—*really* learned—when my son saw me as a hero. His loving perspective allowed me to replace old, worn-out self-judging stories with stories of love. This is now how I evaluate *all* my life stories. Through this lens I scrutinize how I see the facts of my life—do I keep love as my boss, or do I sink to blame, shame, and guilt? I remember that love always ennobles, never judges.

And through the lens of love, I evaluate my future stories and actions. Does this decision support love? Does this course of action serve love and connection, or does it serve fear? Those are the only questions you need answers to as you move forward on your journey.

Life School Point of View (POV)

The Life School POV is a powerful tool to remind us that all the events of our lives have made us exactly who we are today. The person we love and are satisfied with. Or the person who needs some work—but without the Life School POV would never realize this. Not that those events were somehow preordained, but they are all available to us to derive meaning and foster strength and wisdom.

Even the bad—traumatizing and painful—stuff has shaped us into who we are today. It's led us to create resources to support us, to call in help and love that have amazed us when they arrived and filled us with wisdom that has strengthened us for the rest of our lives.

The Life School POV doesn't let us sink into the passive position of being the victim of our circumstances. We make sense out of it—we learn, we grow, we rise. We drop all blame and excuses. This life is ours, plain and simple. We claim full responsibility for all of it. There is no other path to sustainable healing.

You Need a New Story—Let's Write You One!

You feel stuck. You're filled with questions. Now where do you go? How do you reckon with those stories that put the brakes on your healing and make you suffer?

Each story, at its core, involves a false notion or assumption that must be discovered and transformed.

In my hero story I made the false assumption that events of my life were about me—that I was abandoned, unwanted, unworthy. On the surface it looked like that. This concrete and inherently limited perspective of a young person engendered guilt and a very profound sense of unworthiness.

However, with my adult perspective, by using my new tools, the lens of love and the Life School POV, I realized how those events and the actions of others had nothing whatsoever to do with me. It wasn't personal. Their behavior was about them. And I saw that every one of those events shaped me into who I am today. I have unique qualities, perspectives, and wisdom that I could not otherwise have. I gained from those events. And had they been another way, I may have lost what I have now that I so highly value.

These perspectives released the story of abandonment to one of freedom. See how that works?

STORY MINING PRACTICE

Start Here—Sit Down, Get Quiet, Be Present

You are important. Stepping up to change requires your full, reverent attention. Get quiet, relaxed, and focused on the task at hand. Have paper and pen ready. Breathe. Let go of distractions. Soften. Be in your strong center.

Express Gratitude

This puts you on the fast track to success. It instantaneously shifts you into a state of hope and infinite possibilities. It calls in the resources of your great mind, your inner wisdom, and the larger Universe to help you.

Thank you for this challenge, for the opportunity to explore and discover myself, for the growth and freedom that are mine to claim through my honesty and effort. I am grateful.

Clearly State Your Current Story (What's Your Problem or Aspiration?)

Where do you feel stuck? Write this down as your problem, issue, or aspiration. Keep it simple. Don't overthink—write these down quickly.

HEAL KARYN SHANKS MD

- *I am tired all the time.*

- *I am sick and hopeless.*

Decide to Change—Accept Ownership of Your Story

This is your declaration that the problem exists, that you are stuck, and that you claim full ownership of the present circumstances and all that is required to change it.

Ownership means that when *we* are stuck, it's about *us*. By accepting personal responsibility for our story, we facilitate hope: *if it's ours to manage, we can do something about it.* Even when our problems involve others, we can accept responsibility for our part. This releases blame, creating space for others to participate.

Boldly declare your decision to change and claim full responsibility for your problem and its resolution. Contemplate how you create, perpetuate, or fail to facilitate correcting your problem.

- *I sleep only four hours at night because I don't have time to sleep.*

- *This is why I'm tired. I'm committed to creating more time for sleep.*

- *I don't see a way out and have given up on myself.*

- *I have dug myself into a hole (starting with my stories) and am committed to helping myself climb out.*

Story Shifting: Transform Your Problem into a Positive Personal Affirmation

New stories need new neural networks. We can ignite the energy of neuroplasticity by nourishing our brains with new stories. Stories that tell us the truth that our problems can change.

Create a positive, present tense affirmation to articulate your goal. This makes it "sticky," mobilizing the resources needed to bring it to life. It affirms the direction you are headed (forward, into needed change), the possibility of change (away from the perception of being stuck), and attracts the help you need.

- *I enjoy radiant new energy.*

- *I have all the time I need for deep, restorative sleep.*

- *I choose hope.*

- *I receive all the support and resources I need to attain vibrant energy.*

The Moment of Reckoning

If you know what the obstacles to achieving your goal are, why don't you just remove them? If you know you need more sleep, why don't you get more sleep? If you know you need to ask for help, why don't you just do that? What supports those obstacles? What story is present that makes the obstacles necessary? What fears exist?

- *I sleep only four hours at night because I feel I have to do it all—work full time, take care of the kids, do all the household chores, be the ideal spouse—there's no time left for sleep.*

- *I don't deserve to rest or take care of myself. If I do, then I feel guilty.*

- *If I take care of myself, others will suffer because of it.*

- *I have been to many doctors, and they say there are no answers for me.*

What are your obstacles to change? What are your stories? Reflect on this very honestly. Write swiftly and don't overthink.

Take a Time Out

Before continuing, let's shake this out. For some of you this process has been a breeze. By all means, carry on if you wish. For many of us, the problems we have chosen to work on are quite difficult, intense, or bring up challenging emotions. These may be areas in which

we have felt quite stuck, or where we bring up a lot of self-judgment. So, let's take a quick
break to get out of our heads and back into our bodies. Stand up and move. Feel your feet
against the floor. Walk around. Make a cup of tea or get some water. Breathe deeply. Sigh
it out loudly. Let it all go.

Name the False Notion or Assumption in Your Story

You now have a positive personal affirmation that clearly states your goal and the positive change you would like to experience. You also have a problem statement with a story that explains why the problem exists. Recall what those are now.

Now, consider how these statements are at odds with one another. On the one hand you have an exciting new positive affirmation that can energize your movement toward change. On the other hand, there is an essential story about what will happen if that change occurs, that drives your problem and keeps you stuck. These need to be reckoned with.

Look closely at your reasons for staying stuck. What keeps your old story alive? Is it based on the facts of your life? Does it pass scrutiny through the lens of love or the Life School POV?

What do you believe about the outcome if your desired change were to take place? What are you afraid of? What is the worst-case scenario? Are you waiting for support that hasn't come (money, knowledge)? Do you need permission? Are you worried about what people will think? Or of standing alone?

Regardless of what your obstacle is, ultimately only fear stands in your way. In their book, *How the Way We Talk Can Change the Way We Work*, Robert Kegan and Lisa Laskow refer to these fears as the "competing commitments" that serve as our obstacles to successful change. On the one hand we are committed to the change we want. But on the other hand, perhaps unconsciously, we're also committed to protecting ourselves from the harm we perceive will accompany that change.

State Your Fears:

- I sleep only four hours at night because I feel that I have to do it all: work full time, raise the kids, do all the household chores, be the ideal spouse.
  If I don't accomplish all of this, I will be thought of as a failure. If I don't accomplish all of this, I will be a disappointment to someone (to my family, my community, my culture).

- If I take care of myself, others will suffer.
  If I take care of myself, I will shine and those around me (family, friends) will feel resentful or jealous. If I take care of myself my health and energy will soar, I will lead a happier life and my friends in misery will feel abandoned. (Who am I to feel good when everyone else in my life suffers?)

- I have been to many doctors and there are simply no answers for me.
  I am shy and worried about speaking up with my doctors. If I become self-reliant and ask for help, I will be thought of as uppity. I will step on toes. People will be angry with me.

Look carefully at what you've written. Is it at all possible that you've made assumptions here? Are they supported by all the facts?

Do your assumptions pass the scrutiny of the lens of love? The Life School POV?

If there are even hints of doubt, blame, shame, or judgment, consider them to be false notions and assumptions to be discredited and consciously corrected. This is not an easy task and may take you way out of your comfort zone. But it's the truth, and it's your fast track to freedom, energy, and healing.

Practice Courage

Now, ignite your new path with *courage*! Change can and most likely will trigger anxiety, trepidation, or resistance. Expect this and prepare for it.

It is now time to put your new goal and the healthier, more ennobling life story that supports it into practice. Think of it like a scientist: test your hypothesis. This is the step where you muster up courage and go forth into that terra incognita. It's okay to *feel* afraid but resist your fearful *stories*.

Reframe how you think about the fear by assigning new words to describe the physical aspects of fear—the nervousness, racing heart, shortness of breath, frantic thoughts. Like,

"Oh, it feels like anxiety but perhaps that's just my body ramping up for action to support me." Or, *"I'm excited about what's to come."* Don't worry about believing what you say, just practice it. Select your words carefully to support your *decision* to take action with courage.

Practice Your Story

Almost there. Remember? What you *do* is your story. Now that you are ready and supercharged with courage, name your first action step. What are you ready for? The moon? Or, how about baby steps? Keep it small and doable and practice daily. It might look like this:

- *Tonight, I will go to bed early and make sure I get eight hours of sleep. I will do this every night and ask for my family's support.*

- *I will find a Functional Medicine doctor in my community and call for an appointment today.*

- *I will not give up on my healing. I deserve to be well. I will continue to explore resources until my needs are met. I remain resolutely optimistic. I'm in this for the long haul.*

Practice Patience

If you're like me, you want to go fast and take giant leaps right away. We're determined, we're committed, we're excited! We want to move forward, quickly building on our successes and feeling the powerful intoxicating rush of success. But this isn't a race. This is life. Remember, the goal is to build a strong foundation, one that supports our core, our goals, our futures. Big quick wins are exciting, but they're generally not sustainable. They don't have the automaticity that comes with time or the internalization that comes with repetition. No great medieval cathedral was ever built on just a bunch of soaring arches or grandiose facades. There is always a foundation of small bricks, carefully placed, one next to another, one supporting another. Only on that foundation could a cathedral reach to the heavens. And that takes time.

Finally, Embrace Failure as a True Great Teacher

We can be fragile when we are suffering, working hard on healing, and challenged with changes that scare us. It is important to be kind and gentle with ourselves as we do our work. We must expect that there will be setbacks, disappointments, as well as outright miserable failures. We may feel like we've let ourselves down, let others down, totally messed things up, and are now totally stuck for sure!

Fine. Let it be. Roadblocks and disappointments are the inevitable price for being curious and courageous. And just like small children, after we fall down and maybe cry (or drop an f-bomb), we brush ourselves off and stand back up. We giggle as we shake it off. And we take note of what just happened.

Failure invites us to listen and learn. Then try again. That's all. No magic. No bravado. Just Life School.

- *Dang it! I didn't get to bed until midnight again, ugh! I was too ambitious at first. I was getting just four hours of sleep. Tonight, I will shoot for five instead of eight.*

- *I saw a new doctor and was told there is nothing wrong with me yet again. I feel discouraged, but I promised not to give up. I will practice hope and optimism, though it is very hard, and reach out to some friends for advice about how to proceed. I will not give up.*

LAST THOUGHTS

We've come a long way on our journey so far. We've made amazing progress—even if you don't feel it, believe me, you have! We've nourished ourselves with healing space, with love, with a strong center in the face of challenge, with sleep, with movement, and with healthy food. Now we're strengthened by the guiding perspectives of love (the lens of love) and learning (the Life School POV) as we acknowledge, face, and rewrite our stories. All this work is the passage to grace and freedom in our lives. And it's the anchor we need as we venture into the wild realm of the emotions—the *flow* of the deepest, truest wisdom of our souls. Coming up next!

Chapter Nine

FLOW

Trust Your Emotional Wisdom
(Find Your Truth)

Now spacious, nourished, strong in our core, and savvy with our stories, we're prepared to enjoy—and brave—our feelings. The flow of our deepest selves, our emotional genius.

Emotions lay bare the truth that is within us. The truth that cannot be denied. The truth that will find its way—like the irrepressible rivers running wild through the countryside—into our consciousness against all resistance.

So, welcome them—all of them—as your dearest friends. Do not be afraid. Do not judge. They're here for you. Even the feelings that bite and scare are your teachers. Always healing. Always on your side.

EMOTIONS—THE FLOW OF LIFE

The flow of life. That's why we're all here. That's what we aspire to: strength, buoyance, presence . . . ourselves. Emotions are the current of this flow, the rhythm of our interior lives. Carried by primordial waves of energy, our feelings bring us the innate, intuitive, primal, noncognitive wisdom we must have to decode our lives, to grow, and to survive.

While often pleasing and exhilarating, our emotions can also confuse and befuddle us, scare and destabilize us. Our feelings—the ways we instinctively perceive and discern our world—are also what make life seem so hard!

Now, pause here. Breathe. Tap into your strong center. Breathe into your core and feel your strength. Be present right here, in your body. We're entering territory that may feel treacherous. But we're born to do this. We've come prepared.

Emotions deliver information about the state of our lives. This pure, spontaneous perceptual intelligence arises from within our bodies to teach us what we must know about all our experiences. Emotions are liquid insights about the people, the environment, and the conditions of our surroundings. They are the truth within us.

Nothing exhilarates or challenges us quite like what we feel. But for the challenges, it's not really our emotions themselves that throw us off. No, it's the stories we tell about them that twist their true meaning. How we judge and condemn them, shut them down, and fail to understand their unadulterated truth.

It's absolutely critical to our own emotional intelligence to understand that our emotions are not *us*. What throws us off balance and makes life seem so hard, is how we identify ourselves *as* our emotions (*I am guilty, I am unlovable*), rather than as the witness to them (*I feel guilty, I feel unlovable*). Only as the witness, are we prepared to receive what we need to know.

In no other arena of our lives are we asked to be so brave in calling our power back. To step up to our feelings. To feel. Then let go of the tenacious stories that blame, belittle, and deny our true wisdom.

Yes, we feel. We know.

Breathe deeply. Trust your strong center, your anchor. Let's explore what our emotions have to teach us. To do this we must be present within our bodies.

We *Must* Feel

We have to show up for this flow of life we aspire to. We want it. We crave it. But there's a price.

To *really* show up, we've got to go slow and pay attention.

And when we go slow and *really* pay attention, we feel.

No longer will the intensity and distraction of our fast-paced lives block us from feeling. This is our challenge, perhaps the greatest challenge of our lives: to allow ourselves to experience the full range of our emotions and learn to trust the wisdom and intelligence they deliver.

But I Do Feel

"But I *do* feel," you say. You're probably like so many of us—yes, we do feel, but we've learned to control and restrict our feelings, choosing only what's pleasing and comfortable, not scary.

After all, why would we want to feel bad or scared?

With Joy Comes Pain

But the problem is that we can't choose one without the other. When we shove down pain, we also lose joy. The best we can do is some lukewarm approximation of the true glory that is possible. Our emotional censorship invariably comes with that price.

But by showing up, going slow, and paying attention, we get it all: truly feeling. The suffering that is our genius, that brings the truth, that leads to mind-blowing transformation. The joy that lifts us up and lights the world.

Yes, We'll Squirm

Feeling will inevitably take us into discomfort we'd rather avoid. Feeling *will* make us squirm, *will* make us suffer, *will* ask us to face up to difficult truths.

Feeling is the Only Path to Growth

But feeling is the only path to deep learning and discovery of ourselves. It's the only path to growth. It's the only path to the grace and magic of our humanness. It's our connection to the people and world around us. We must have our emotional genius to be in the true flow of our lives.

Isabella's Emotional Healing

Isabella is a fellow physician with a busy practice. When she first came to see me, she was suffering from severe fatigue, migraine headaches, and achy, stiff muscles. She was also intensely irritable and intermittently resentful and angry. At thirty-three years old, she considered herself happily married, and was the mother of two smart, active children. She found it challenging to manage her busy life.

Her emotional symptoms seemed to escalate every month just before her period started. Each month, as she passed the midpoint of her menstrual cycle, she would feel the dreaded tension build, reaching a crescendo a few days prior to her period onset, when she would feel intense frustration, time pressure, and rage toward what she believed were little things. She was exhausted, achy, and anxious. She felt disabled by her physical symptoms and bewildered by her powerful emotions.

As she told me her story, she sobbed. She felt helpless to the power of her emotions, ashamed for how she felt, and completely out of control. She described herself as "a monster" for a week out of every month. She never acted out her anger in abusive ways, but she believed that her deeply troubling emotions were something *wrong with her*. How could she possibly feel such anger and frustration when her life was so blessed? She felt like a failure for having them. Eventually, these feelings would subside, and she would tuck her concerns away until the next month when they would arise again.

As we explored her story, many contributing elements came to light. First of all, she was sleep deprived. She was frequently awakened by her children, and she was always the one to get up with them in the night. She routinely went to bed late, after the household chores were completed, and got up early to get herself and kids ready for the day. She picked them up from school in the afternoon, helped with homework, drove them to their activities, got supper ready for the family, then managed baths, story time, and tucking them into bed. Her husband came home from work around six, enjoyed supper and family time, then retreated to his study before going to bed. Essentially Isabella took care of the family and household duties on her own, in addition to working full time. In the telling of this story, her fury and resentment were palpable. Something had to give.

When I asked her if she had ever spoken to her husband about how she felt, she looked at me, stunned, and said no. She explained that she didn't want to burden him after he worked hard all day. Isabella did not realize that it was not necessarily all up to her to take care of everyone and everything. Intellectually she felt like she was a modern woman who could partner with her husband to share the duties of taking care of the family and house. But once the kids came along, she jumped in, without thinking it through, and took over the role of sole caretaker.

Our priority was to deal with her unresolved anger and frustration about the division of labor within the household between herself and her husband. This was driving much of her distress and fueled her physical symptoms. Because women tend to be more tuned in to their emotions during the second half of their menstrual cycle, it was no surprise that Isabella's powerful emotions, that she otherwise tried to suppress, would come up each month to hit her between the eyes, warning her that her life was seriously out of balance. But she didn't see that. She saw herself being a "monster."

She literally internalized her anger. The physical stress of repressing these powerful emotions resulted in profound physical and emotional symptoms. For Isabella, anger and frustration were taboo when she had so many blessings in her life. Instead of listening to what her emotions had to say to her, she felt guilty for having them, worked hard to push them away, then shamed for the tsunami of rage that struck each month.

Isabella spoke with her husband about how she was feeling, and while he was surprised because it had never come up, he agreed to help out. He had assumed she wanted to take care of everything and went along with it but admitted that he'd actually wished he could participate more in bath time and reading bedtime stories. She always jumped in and did it, and he was too frightened by her anger to question it. They divided up supper duty, bath time, and reading stories. He started doing more food prep and helping to clean up after supper. They hired a housekeeper to come in weekly to do the major household cleaning. She also cut back on her work hours a bit so she would have more time for the self-care she badly needed.

Isabella's tension eased substantially. She had trouble letting go of her well-practiced tendency to jump in and control everything in her life, and still felt a ramping up of irritability at the end of her cycle, but it became much less intense as she became acquainted with the true messages her body was sending her through her emotions: that she needed to be less vigilant about everything, to claim better boundaries for herself, to ask for help, and leave room in her life for herself.

Isabella's powerful emotions and the sensations and symptoms of her body taught her profound lessons.

Thought Exercise: Isabella

Imagine how Isabella was feeling—the frustration of an "unsolvable" situation. Powerful feelings about emotions she would not allow herself to acknowledge. Can you relate? How would you advise her?

Lessons from Isabella

- Emotions are physical, with physical sensations and consequences.

- Emotions convey wisdom and information about our lives. Isabella's were warning her about her imbalanced life and exhaustion—her loss of a strong center.

- When we ignore the messages of our emotions, they will amplify themselves to get our attention. Repressed long enough, they will lead to physical symptoms, imbalances, and illness, as Isabella's did.

- We judge our emotions (which are really value neutral) as "good" or "bad," creating stories and distorting their true meaning. Isabella felt like a monster for experiencing the rage that was just the messenger arriving to warn her about what did not work in her life.

- We misconstrue our stories about our emotions for the emotions themselves: "I feel like a monster," rather than, "I feel angry, what's going on?" "I'm out of control," rather than, "My life feels out of control." "Something is wrong with me," rather than, "What do these uncomfortable emotions have to teach me about what's not working in my life?"

- Paying attention and heeding the messages of our emotions leads us to self-discovery, transformation, and freedom. Isabella's work with her powerful emotions led to both emotional and physical healing.

EMOTIONS ARE IN THE BODY

Emotions have a biology—energy, electricity, and biochemistry that are physical. As such, emotions and how we experience them are affected by the strength, resilience, and dynamic balance we create within our bodies (as we explored in chapter four). Emotional biology—neurochemicals, stress and energy molecules, immune cell response, physical sensations, movement, and behavior—changes with our bodies' dynamic state of health and equilibrium. Therefore, we can shift our point of equilibrium, our emotional balance, and our emotional *experience* through how we care for our bodies.

Sound like hocus-pocus? From your own everyday experiences, you know it's not. Remember how good you felt last time you had a great night's sleep, waking well rested and restored? How the day was brighter? How your step was a bit lighter? How there was simply more positive potential to the day? Or how at the end of a long, tiring day, you felt less happy, more anxious, and more irritable? How about persistent pain and the loneliness and despair that can come with it? Or prolonged suffering and hopelessness? These are all examples of the body-mind-emotion connection in operation. Understanding this integration allows us to use our bodies as key inroads to emotional awareness and intelligence. Our bodies are how we can actively direct our emotional lives.

Self-care, using the foundational strategies we've explored throughout this book, is essential to this work. The scientific literature bearing this out is packed to the brim with studies confirming the connection between health and emotions. For instance, immune cell activation, the basis of inflammation, always affects how we feel. It's common to feel depressed or despairing when we're sick with the flu—our emotional biology and our emotional experience are affected by the intense inflammation that results from the viral infection and activation of our immune cells. The same is true for chronic infections and persistent inflammatory or autoimmune conditions. Resolving the underlying inflammatory immune dysfunction and creating body resilience through self-care leads to remarkable improvements in how we feel and behave as energy recovers and the body heals. And it also feeds back—as people emotionally feel better, inflammation is decreased. I see this in my practice every day.

Being *in* our bodies is part of the path to understanding our emotions. Our bodies connect us in present-moment awareness. All the work we've done to find, nourish, protect, and challenge our strong center—to become present within our bodies—is how we show up for our emotions. It's how we anchor ourselves within when the current gets strong. And it's how we go with the flow of our lives.

THE EMOTIONAL REALM IS TRICKY—TRUTH, INTUITIVE GUIDANCE, AND THE INTELLIGENCE OF THE BODY

Enter the realm of the emotions. They're wild. Spontaneous. Unpredictable. Forces to be reckoned with, they find their way into our consciousness in spite of our best efforts to shove them away, numb them out, or deny them. That can be scary! Why? They bring us the truth. Truth we may not want. Truth that may disrupt the comfortable status quo of our lives. Be warned—but also celebrate—that emotions represent the energy of our deepest wisdom.

We must become savvy about the common ways we manage discomfort about our emotional truths: how we tame them, blame them, numb them, disconnect from them by playing "nice," and polarize them into "good versus bad." We must call back our truth, intuitive guidance, and intelligence of the body. Our power.

We Tame Emotions

We're taught to tame our emotions from an early age. In our culture we downplay the value of our emotions in favor of the more factual, logical, and rational inputs of our minds. We fear emotions' raw, wild, and untamed nature and how they might lead us to danger and destruction. We fear their power and unpredictability. We fear the way they operate outside the bounds of our conscious control. We are trained to resist, control, and cast them off, but this leads to the loss of emotional intelligence.

We Blame Emotions

Emotional information is very pure, but our lack of emotional fluency makes them seem cryptic and difficult to understand. Because our logical brains don't always trust our emotions, we scrutinize them with deep skepticism, *interpreting* their meaning through rules and rationality, and disbelieving them when they don't tell us what we want to hear. By filtering our emotions through our dominant intellects we lose the nuance of their raw data. We see them, instead, through our stories—engendering blame, judgment, fear, shame, guilt, mistrust, and confusion. We all know these stories: "It's all my fault." "It's all your fault." "I don't belong." "I'm a terrible person." "I'm crazy."

We Numb Emotions

We're terrified to feel our "negative" (yet entirely normal) emotions. Fear, guilt, shame, anger, and jealousy are particularly scary. We numb ourselves to them in the many creative ways we know all too well: perfectionism (we're never enough), excessive work (idle hands are the devil's playground), compulsive, pleasure-seeking behaviors (like shopping, gaming, social media, sex, television watching, gambling, and so forth), drugs (alcohol, stimulants, sedatives, opiates), or adrenaline-seeking behavior (going fast, creating drama, gossip, danger).

We're Nice

On the other end of the spectrum, we become obsessed with experiencing only "positive" emotions. We do this through addiction to exhilaration, seeking experiences to engender connection, excitement, and bliss, even when we're not genuinely feeling them. Or we may only allow positive emotions, so we force them—we act "nice," pretending things are good when they're not.

This is not to say that we shouldn't cultivate positive emotions, like love and gratitude, or act with kindness, empathy, and compassion toward others. We need strong neural networks for love, and our relationships, communities, and planet need more kindness and empathy. But life and the world aren't all good. We need to know and accept that. Our emotions bring us this essential wisdom from all our experiences, which we use to learn, and make discerning and wise choices.

Nice is distinct from kindness, compassion, and empathy. Nice is dangerous. Nice disguises our authenticity. Nice shuts us down and shuts others down. It keeps our relationships, interactions, and experiences superficial by closing the door to the truth we all desperately need. Truth that must be heard and will find its way in, one way or another—like the anger, resentment, and jealousy that Isabella felt. We've all been there. We all know this.

We Polarize Emotions: Good versus Bad

Our discomfort with the subterranean energy of our emotions leads to polarizing them as "good versus bad." But emotions themselves are value neutral, so these judgments only apply to the stories we tell about them. Many of these "good versus bad" stories are learned from our families and tribes. They're born from anxiety about the intensity of the emotions, concern for our stability and survival, and fear about grappling honestly with what's not working.

Some of these stories are about power. The family structures and social institutions we're born into are often built on outdated notions of power—their dogmatic, hierarchical foundations deny and disempower true feelings seen as threats to the status quo. In this way, many of our voices, experiences, and innate wisdom are crushed through the "good versus bad" story. That means we lose this precious resource that would help us understand ourselves better, grow wiser, and strengthen our social structures.

But That's Not Us

None of this is us. None of this is what we aspire to. We've shown up here for a different experience. We're changing and going after our true potential. We're rising up. We're healing. We're stepping over those social and tribal ideas that stifle us. We're claiming our emotions as our own, as our birthright, as the wisdom within us. We're removing the value judgments and inviting it all. No more nice. No more dishonesty. We've built a strong center. From this core we have the strength to reckon with *all* our emotional wisdom.

Permission Slip: Permission to Feel

"I am so blessed by so much in my life, but I feel miserable."

"I've accomplished so much in my life, but I never feel like I'm enough."

"Everyone loves him, but he makes me feel uncomfortable."

"If I speak up about what I feel, I will be persecuted."

"I am suffering, and feel I have no right to."

"I am in pain, and for this I feel shame."

So many feelings! Too many of these feelings we judge ourselves for and feel uncomfortable about, letting them drive us to complete distraction.

If we go slow, we will feel.

Going fast is often a strategy we use (often unconsciously) not to feel. For example: If I go fast, striving for more and more accomplishment and success, I may not realize that guilt and shame are what drive me. I know I'm never satisfied, but I just keep going. By going slow and paying attention to my feelings, I get close to them. I feel them. I feel the guilt and shame for not being enough. Feelings that are never sufficiently soothed by the hard work I do. When I slow down, I come face to face with the truth that drives me. To claim my freedom, I must reckon with these feelings. To reclaim my present-moment life I must slow down, stop working so hard, and feel.

See how that works? Once more, we're called to action—to show up, go slow, and pay attention. We can passively live our emotional lives and never know who we are, or we can actively call our power back, feel our feelings, and step into their sacred knowledge and freedom.

We start with permission to feel. Remember our other permission slips? Let's write another one:

Dear [your name here],

You have my full permission to be your whole, true self, with all your feelings. Every. Last. One. All your feelings are sacred, essential parts of you. Each one will tell you something you must know to help you heal, to help you become whole, to lead you to freedom.

Let your feelings be exactly what they are. Let them flow. Let the uncomfortable ones have their space. You must hear them all!

And remember, you are not your feelings. You are awareness. You are the simple presence that sees and feels. The witness. The compassionate observer. Breathe into this knowledge and slow it all down. Be in your body and breathe.

No shame. No guilt. No need to hide. Only love. Let those sacred feelings fly. Let them rise up and be your truth. Let us look at them in the light of day and find the beautiful truth of who you are. For whatever you feel, no matter how dark, lonely, or lost, you are also love. However you may be suffering, you are love. You have my permission to do this. And I will always be at your side. Protecting you. Cheering you on.

Love, Me.

THE PHYSICS OF EMOTIONS

"We are wired for bliss."

—*Candace Pert, Molecules of Emotion*

I find it helpful to understand the physics of emotions because it helps relieve the burden of feeling helpless to them. It gives us a framework for working with them in a direct and less threatening way, bypassing our endless stories and judgments.

To work with our emotions, we must get into our bodies. This calls us to be *in* our bodies. Remember our exploration of embodiment in chapter six? Embodiment empowers us through real-time connection to emotional energy.

Emotional Flow

Just like the flow of chemicals and electricity in our biochemical pathways, emotions create real electrochemical charges within the body that give them the fluidity and movement we associate with their experience. We can all relate to this flow aspect of our emotions as they expand or contract within us—we feel them physically. Great love or tremendous grief literally rocks our insides. Exuberance lifts us up off our feet.

Emotional Geography

Further, we experience emotions regionally. We can feel where emotions tend to localize within our bodies—like love and grief in our chests, or guilt and shame in our guts. We sense the expansion of powerful emotions like anger, perhaps rising up in the midsection, then quickly compressing the body, contracting muscles, inhibiting breathing, focusing attention, and possibly mobilizing us into action. Or awe: how those amazing sunsets, shooting stars, or heroic actions seem to explode all through us. Yes, we can all sense the physical locality, movement, and power of our emotions.

Emotional Vibration

In addition to their localizing tendency, the electricity of emotions confers a vibration that is unique to the quality and intensity of the emotion being experienced. For instance, love and gratitude have high vibrational frequencies that we can feel, which lift us up and energize us. In contrast, lower vibration emotions, like frustration and anger, make us feel subdued, contracted, and tense.

This vibrational quality of our emotions is what allows us to feel the emotions of others, even without speaking. We've all felt this, how when we walk into a room where people are happy, loving, and welcoming versus angry, we pick up on different vibrations—it's a real sensory experience that we all understand instantly. We know exactly how we feel around them—and how *they* feel—without exchanging words. We feel the electrical energy of the emotions.

Emotional Resonance

Our attunement to the emotional energy of others is simple physics. This phenomenon, which we call resonance, is how we are able to know immediately, when in the presence of someone, whether we like them or not. Whether we feel comfortable around them. Whether they like us. There are people with whom we feel elevated and alive. With others we feel depleted and exhausted. We instinctively sense their emotional vibrational energy even if we are not consciously aware of it.

This vibrational quality of our emotions is part of the inner wisdom of "gut" feelings, hunches, impulses, and intuition. It's how we attract what we need and repel what we don't. It's what creates that unspoken connection that we experience with the people in our lives. And it's a huge part of what creates our mood and our energy.

We are particularly sensitive to being elevated by positive, high vibrational emotions. As Candace Pert says, "We're wired for bliss." There is a large body of science that demonstrates the myriad positive effects on our physiology, behavior, and mood as a result of exposure to positive emotions. We learn and think better. Our health is better. We are less depressed and anxious. We have more energy and vibrancy.

Emotional Sensing: Intuition and Empathy

Though we are all able to process the sensations of emotional information, we are constitutionally different in how our bodies do so. We're each uniquely neurologically wired at birth with regard to how we take in sensory information. For example, some of us—particularly introverts—are more sensitive to this energetic information. We also all learn differently and acquire different skill sets for thinking and feeling. While all of us have access to the emotional energy within and around us, for some of us this energy is more readily available.

On the high end of this sensitivity spectrum are people we refer to as intuitive empaths. These people are exquisitely sensitive to emotional-energetic information. They are particularly tuned in to the energy around them, feeling it in their bodies. While this form of emotional awareness can be a gift, it is also fraught with challenges. Many intuitive empaths don't understand the nature of their feelings. They may mistake the sensations from others' emotions as their own and can become easily overwhelmed by them. Many empaths find it difficult to be in crowds or groups of people because of the overwhelming onslaught of energetic information, and they become easily exhausted or anxious. They need quiet, restorative time to clear out and recover. The challenge for intuitive empaths is to sort out the emotional information all around them while protecting themselves from overload.

Others are less attuned to the subtle emotional energy of the body, having a more dominant intellect-centered connection to emotional information. Being more concrete and rational, they are better at understanding action and verbally expressed emotions. They may not be as adept as intuitive empaths at picking up on emotional energy when it is not expressed to them in a tangible form. However, just as empaths can learn to protect themselves from the energy all around them, head-centered people can learn to tune in.

EMOTIONAL ORGANIZATION WITHIN THE BODY

Emotions are anatomically organized through the body. We know this through awareness of emotions and their tendency to localize regionally within the body. Emotional anatomy is part of the emotional fluency that assists us in working with emotions directly and constructively.

Traditional and Modern Ideas of Emotional Anatomy

According to ancient Hindu tradition, there are seven major emotional energy centers within the body, referred to as chakras, *cakra* in Sanskrit, meaning "wheel." These centers represent meeting points, or nodes, for the channels that carry our life force energy, each associated with particular emotions. Chakras were first written about in the Vedas, the oldest written tradition in India (1500-500 BC), recorded from oral tradition by Brahmins.

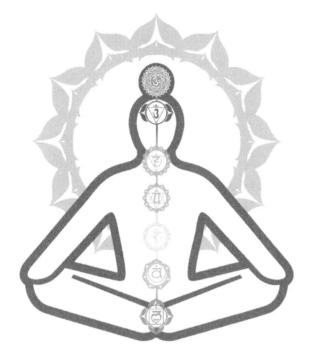

Vedic Chakra System

CROWN
Connection to Divine, Universal Intelligence

THIRD EYE
Wisdom, Discernment

THROAT
Verbal Expression, Listening

HEART CENTER
Love, Compassion

SOLAR PLEXUS
Personal Power, Self-Worth

PELVIS
Creativity, Pleasure, Personal Boundaries

ROOT
Survival, Belonging, Nourishment

This ancient description of the emotional anatomy of the body aligns closely with a modern counterpart—the construct of human emotional developmental hierarchy popularized by Abraham Maslow, the well-known psychologist, in the 1940's. Without any indication that he was aware of the Vedic chakra system, he created Maslow's hierarchy of (emotional) needs, which looks much like what the Hindus described, and is the basis for modern psychology and how we understand emotional development even today.

At the base of Maslow's pyramidal-shaped Hierarchy of Needs are those emotional needs and experiences that are necessary for survival, which must be tended to first, before the higher levels become accessible. We have to feel safe and able to nourish ourselves in the most basic ways before we can devote energy to other aspects of life.

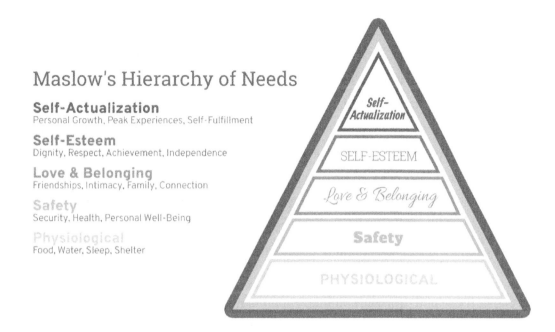

Maslow's Hierarchy of Needs

Self-Actualization
Personal Growth, Peak Experiences, Self-Fulfillment

Self-Esteem
Dignity, Respect, Achievement, Independence

Love & Belonging
Friendships, Intimacy, Family, Connection

Safety
Security, Health, Personal Well-Being

Physiological
Food, Water, Sleep, Shelter

Located in the middle section of Maslow's pyramid is love and belonging, analogous to the centrally located heart center in the Vedic Chakra system. This is the central hub in both traditions, representing love, gratitude, and deep intuitive wisdom. Toward the top of the pyramid are higher functions associated with self-esteem and self-actualization, which depend on the maturity and full expression of all levels below.

While Maslow didn't intend for his pyramidal-shaped hierarchy of needs to represent the human body, if you examine it side-by-side with the chakra system, you can see it is closely aligned with the Vedic anatomical construct, and reveals our more modern understanding of body-mind integration. The two systems reveal the same progression and organization.

Both these venerable traditions show that emotional development, maturity, and balance depend on meeting our physiological and survival needs first. Beyond that, full emotional maturity and potential depends on integration and expression of all the emotions within the body: associated with safety, power, relationships, self-esteem, love, voice, intuition, and connection to a higher power.

WORK WITH THE BODY'S EMOTIONAL ROADMAP

The emotional anatomy of the body guides us in our pursuit of understanding our emotional intelligence. It shows us where our emotions are expressed within the body. There aren't well-defined separations between the emotional centers of the body, but they are loosely organized according to the structures described by the Vedic chakra system and Maslow's hierarchy of needs. In the construct of emotional anatomy that I present to you, I've favored the use of seven emotional centers like the Vedic model, rather than the five of Maslow's, as they allow for more depth of exploration of the range of human emotions.

While this system and way of thinking about the emotions as having a geography within the body may be unfamiliar to you, I ask you to take this journey with me. In my experience it's helpful to become familiar with this emotional roadmap because the regional physical attributes of the emotions invite targeted awareness and swift intervention.

We often make more progress when we work with our emotions through the body because it allows us to bypass our stories and judgments about them. Working with emotional energy in a physical way supports us as witnesses to the value-neutral information they contain.

Finally, because the emotions reside within the body, they will be healthiest when we're healthy: well rested; well nourished; balanced, and mobile; strong and present within our core centers; and fully engaged in present-time awareness.

Emotional imbalances are more likely when the body is depleted of energy, when we're in pain, or when we're actively resisting our feelings.

Our Emotional Foundation

The first three emotional centers span our lower body from toes to solar plexus. This is where our foundational emotions reside, in accordance with the first three Vedic chakras and the physiologic and safety regions of Maslow's hierarchy of needs. These are the centers that support our instinctual drive for survival and personal power—within ourselves, in our relationships, and within our tribes.

When these areas are strong, when the emotions that localize there are allowed full free expression, and when we accept their truth, we tend to feel safe, stable, grounded, connected to our tribe and loved ones, and tuned into our own strength and worth. This is our strong center. These emotional centers are foundational, and they must be strong to support the rest.

First Emotional Center (Root)

This area includes the feet, legs, pelvic floor, and hips. These lower aspects of our bodies make direct connection with the earth, and represent survival, belonging, and nourishment. This is where we experience our essential connection to nature, our tribes, and families. When we're well nourished, safe, and feel like we belong, the first emotional center is strong, leading us to feel stable, secure, connected, and calm. This doesn't mean we have to come from perfect families. We can create a strong root on our own.

Our work in this emotional center is to make sure we feel safe, and to create and affirm strong connections with our people, our communities, the larger world, and all of nature. We must feel this strength and release anxiety.

Exercise: First Emotional Center (Root)

Breathe: Breathe into the root of the body: your feet, legs, base of the pelvis, and hips.

Affirm: All is One. I am safe and protected. I am grounded. The earth supports me.

Move: Allow your feet, without shoes, to experience full contact with the ground. Spend as much time as possible without shoes. This strengthens them and assures your survival-oriented brain that you are standing strong on your own feet. Engage your legs—walk, climb, run. Open your hips—squat, sit on the ground, and receive bodywork.

Second Emotional Center (Pelvis)

This area includes the pelvic bowl (created by the pelvic bones and sacrum) and pelvic organs. This is where we experience passion and essential yearnings as creations of the natural world. Our full expression as human beings and ability to connect and relate to one another in healthy and balanced ways arises from this emotional center. This includes our sexuality, our boundaries within relationships, sense of economic fairness (money), and fertility—both biological and creative, as it relates to how we give birth to our own creative urges. Strength in this center allows us to experience pleasure, to play, to express ourselves creatively, and create healthy boundaries in all of our relationships.

Feelings of guilt or sense of unfairness within our important relationships must be transformed into healthy connections and boundaries. We must generate and give birth to creative expression. We must lighten up and be playful.

Exercise: Second Emotional Center

Breathe: Breathe into the pelvic bowl—the space between your seat and the tops of your hip bones.

Affirm: We honor one another. I create strong personal boundaries. I freely express my true, creative, passionate nature. I live my truth and my purpose.

Move: Walk, feet on the earth, swinging your arms freely, swaying your beautiful hips, playfully and effortlessly releasing into this simple movement. Any playful or freely creative activity (no rules—improvise!) will activate and strengthen this center.

Third Emotional Center (Solar Plexus)

The third emotional center includes the abdomen above the pelvis and extends to the solar plexus, or diaphragm. This is where we experience our emotional sense of self. Our feelings of self-love, self-worth, and personal power are localized here. Shame is the challenge of this center, when we fear existentially that we are not enough just as we are and continuously strive for an imagined perfection. We're called to be our true, authentic selves by this center. We must transform shame into acceptance, forgiveness, and personal empowerment. A strong third emotional center connects us to our true nature as necessary contributors to this world.

Exercise: Third Emotional Center

Breathe: Breathe into the core of the body.

Affirm: I honor myself. I am enough exactly as I am now. I am a blessing to this world. I am my true, whole, authentic self. I love myself.

Move: Engage your core in everything you do. Stand and move with strength from your core center. Build fire here with abdominal crunches, leg lifts, or sitting V-ups. Resist postures that keep you folded forward or covering your core center with your arms.

Fourth Emotional Center (Heart Center)

The fourth emotional center, or heart center, is the hub connecting all the centers above and below. It resides in the center of both the Vedic and Maslow roadmaps. When regularly nourished and strengthened with love and gratitude, it inspires and heals all the other centers. When we use our intentions and positive emotions to activate the emotional energy of the heart, we enjoy improved health and deeper love.

The heart center includes the chest and back as well as the arms and shoulders. It's all about love. When this area is healthy, the energy of love flows out from it in all directions, inspiring and healing the other emotional centers. By activating the heart center with expressions of love (remember the HeartMath research from chapter three?), gratitude, kindness, compassion, and forgiveness, we heal the challenges of this center—grief, isolation, and loneliness. Here, we transform vulnerability into strength, and we feel nourished by our loving connections to others. An important lesson of this center is learning to both give and receive love. The flow of love is the flow of life. It has the power to heal all other emotions.

Exercise: Fourth Emotional Center (Heart Center)

Breathe: Breathe into the center of the chest.

Affirm: I am love. I freely give and receive love. I am grateful. I forgive everything and everyone. I receive universal love. I love myself.

Move: Stand and move with an open heart. Carry your head high, allow your shoulders to rest back in their sockets, straighten your core, and let the light of your heart shine out to the world. Dare to open your chest to receive love. Hug in with your strong shoulders before extending out to others.

The Higher Centers

These are the emotional centers of communication. Where we take in the information of both our inner and outer worlds to create meaningful understanding. There are obstacles here—how do we translate what we learn and experience into practical wisdom, without getting tripped up by our assumptions and stories?

Fifth Emotional Center (Throat)

This center includes the throat and neck. This is where we both speak and hear the truth. It's where we communicate with the world about who we are and what we believe. It's our interface with the world, where we demonstrate how we have been censored or restricted and how we do the same to others. We must allow our voices to permeate the world and carry the truth and the message from our hearts that love is all there is.

While learning to speak our truth, we must also cultivate the strength and presence to stay quiet and listen. Many of us need to learn when it is important to be quiet.

Exercise: Fifth Emotional Center (Throat)

Breathe: Breathe into the throat and neck.

Affirm: I speak and hear the truth. My voice is necessary to this world. I exercise my strength by quietly listening.

Move: Use your voice but also exercise restraint. Speak up about what's on your mind, but also stay quiet and actively listen. Activate your vocal cords by sighing and breathing audibly, humming, and singing. Whistle while you work.

Sixth Emotional Center (Third Eye)

This area between the eyes, referred to as the third eye, is considered to be the seat of our great minds. Will it reveal the truth? Wisdom? Or get us stuck in tenacious stories? When healthy, the sixth emotional center collaborates with the wisdom of the heart and the concentration of the ears to understand and access true knowledge. In the energy of this center, we either commit to our stories (and potential untruths) or to being open minded—embracing mystery and uncertainty (the only *real* truth).

Exercise: Sixth Emotional Center (Third Eye)

Breathe: Breathe into the space between your eyes.

Affirm: I am wise, insightful, intuitive, and discerning. I do my heart's bidding. I know what's true and not true. I soften my stories. I open my mind to infinite possibilities.

Move: Smile with your whole face to soften your mind. Intensely engage your entire body while keeping a soft, relaxed face. Get deeply into your body. Go for a brisk walk, swing your arms freely, and let your mind release its worries, concerns, and judgments.

Seventh Emotional Center (Crown)

According to the chakra tradition, the area at the crown of the head is where we have access to the energy of universal truth and intelligence (God, the Divine, Universal intelligence). Not in a religious sense, but as universal energy available to us all, regardless of how we choose to define it. This energy enters at our apex and permeates our whole being, filling us with wise, healing Divine energy. This eternal source of energy is thought to always be available to us.

Exercise: Seventh Emotional Center (Crown)

Breathe: Breathe into the crown of the head. Breathe in light through the crown, feel that light flow from the crown into the body and flow with the breath into the ground below.

Affirm: I receive the light, love, and healing energy of the Divine Universe. I receive the grace of God. (Choose your own nouns here: for example, Source, Divine Intelligence, Nature.)

Move: Stand strong in a receptive power pose. Stand tall with your bare feet hip-distance apart. Engage your core—thighs back, buttocks and abdominal muscles engaged, pelvis tilted forward. Allow your arms to hang at your sides with shoulders released into their sockets, hands facing forward, heart open. Squeeze your shoulder blades together. Now, tilt your face toward the sky. Open your arms out to the sides of your body or raise them up overhead. You are poised in this position to receive. Be bold and ask for what you need. Keep your heart open and mind soft. Express gratitude. Feel the light. Open to grace.

THE INTELLIGENCE OF NEGATIVE EMOTIONS— NAVIGATING THE STORM

"Not all storms come to disrupt your life. Some come to clear your path."

—*Rumi*

Why are there emotions that make us squirm? What is it about them that feels so uncomfortable?

We have a strong attraction to negativity. Negative information, negative stories, and negative feelings take up a lot of space in our minds. This trait, known as the "negativity bias," is a survival strategy of our brains. We glom on to thoughts, feelings, and experiences posing potential threats, allowing them to take priority space in our minds. This drives a physical stress response, flooding us with energy, anxiety, and discomfort to get our attention and mobilize us to action.

This negativity bias may keep us alive at times, but more often, the negative experiences crowd out the rest—the good and the beautiful. Our negative stories and uncomfortable feelings get way more credit for power and significance than they deserve.

Emotional Navigation: It's All about Balance

But we need *all* our feelings. Good and bad. It's not either/or, good versus bad, brave versus fearful, sad versus happy. No. It's a mess. Our human mess. A mess that, if we're present for it, is the beauty of our lives. We're living real lives. We're challenged. We must be at the helm of our ship, with our hands poised on our ship's rudder, ready to change course as we heed the navigational intelligence of our emotions. Without *all* our emotions, we're just drifting. We're nowhere. We need all our emotions to keep our center strong. To be present. So, let's look at the big ones.

Anger, Rage, and Hate

The energy of anger is powerful. Whether our own or someone else's, it feels unpredictable and dangerous. Where might it lead us? How might it destroy us? We throw anger under the bus, misconstruing it as "meanness," "loss of control," or "irrational." We take the anger of others personally, whether it is directed at us or not.

But anger has a purpose. Anger is about fairness, justice, and where our boundaries have been breached. We must find ways to express this vital information and to receive it with the keen eye of a compassionate observer. Repeatedly denying the message of anger by subjugating ourselves to the control of others, allowing unacceptable circumstances, or casting blame where it doesn't belong, will take its toll. Suppressing anger will always lead to the amplification of its message, escalating to resentment, rage, hatred, explosive behavior, and physical symptoms—fatigue, depression, headaches, and insomnia.

Denying the truth our anger brings leads us to the toxicity of powerlessness and resentment toward others. Denying the truth of others' anger closes the door on them and gets in the way of what we may need to learn about ourselves within those relationships.

Exercise: How Do We Reckon with Anger?

Own it. Know that anger is an entirely normal, necessary, and healthy human emotion. But receive anger as the messenger and don't make it personal—no blame or shame.

Breathe. Tap into your strong center. Soften. Anger will rise up from your strong center to help you see the personal energy, perimeter, and fairness violations that inevitably happen in our everyday lives. Anger is always a call to reflection and action. It doesn't have to be destructive.

Get into your body. Anger rises up from the root and core of the body with strong energy to mobilize us into action. Move your body—walk, run, do yoga, do chores. Get into a power pose—any strong, receptive, open stance. Engage with anger in a positive and constructive way by allowing its energy to move rather than get stuck, escalate, or explode.

Affirm: I am safe. I create strong personal boundaries.

Consider: What does your anger have to say? What's the message?

Fear

Fear, like anger, has been socially maligned and misinterpreted. We've been taught to think feeling scared means we are "weak" or "wimpy." We polarize fear from bravery, thinking we must contain one or the other, rather than both. As a result, fear makes us feel vulnerable, unsafe, inadequate, and easily overwhelmed. We work hard to hide our fear, depleting our energy, and making our lives feel unsafe.

Fear is often a constructive response to real danger, which we should heed for our safety. It is an innate response to change, to feeling uncertain, and taking risks. Fear can be tricky to work with because it comes with the discomfort of stress hormones that heighten our anxiety and trigger our innate impulse to fight or flee. This can muddle our perceptions about what we fear, making it difficult to discern the true message.

Exercise: How Do We Reckon with Fear?

Mark Twain once wrote, "Courage is resistance to fear, mastery of fear—not absence of fear."

So, in that spirit, first step up to fear. Recognize that fear is a call to action. Know that we can be both afraid and brave at the same time. We can be firmly in our strong center and still feel fear.

Breathe. Find your strong center. Breathe here. Feel the strength within you. Feel your courage.

Get into your body. Fear is a call to action but can also be overwhelming and befuddling. We must have a way to manage the intense stress, anxiety, and physical energy that can arrive with fear. Jump right into your body—walk, run, work out, do chores. Become completely engaged in your full-body movement and mental concentration on the task at hand.

Affirm: I am safe. I am strong. I am guided and protected.

Consider: Trust your inner wisdom and guidance. Remember how to recognize heart wisdom from chapter three? Put that into action here. Fear is a teacher, guide, and energy source to power your actions. Ask your fear, "What do you have to teach me?"

Guilt and Shame

We've spoken about guilt and shame before in chapter two—the most toxic of emotions, particularly when allowed to persist. Still, in small doses guilt and shame may be valuable as internal signs that we've done wrong. They get our attention and guide us to take responsibility for our actions, to make amends, to say we're sorry, and to help heal wounds we've caused. The challenge is in claiming our bad deeds, without sliding into the toxic cesspool of guilt and shame.

Persistent guilt and shame are self-condemning stories that sap our strength and stomp on our souls. They're not *our* stories—we've learned them. We've learned how we're to blame for how others have behaved. Or how we're unworthy for not meeting others' expectations. Guilt and shame weaken us in the face of the important work of our lives.

Exercise: How Do We Reckon with Guilt and Shame?

Breathe. Tap into your strong center. Breathe deeply here.

Get into your body. Engage your strong core. Stand straight. Shoulders back. Be in your strong core center. Move or hold your body from this place of strength.

Affirm: I am enough just as I am. I am strong.

Consider: How have you taken others' actions or words personally? What assumptions have you made about yourself that aren't true? What blame, judgment, or social/family "rules" have you unfairly imposed upon yourself? On others?

Know this with absolute certainty: You are enough just as you are. You are love and light. You were born worthy. Period. Nothing that ever happens is personal.

Jealousy

Jealousy. We all know the sting of it and have been smacked down by the shame of it, but it's really a normal part of being humans who thrive on connection. It comes up in a flash, unbidden, and hits us between the eyes. At its worst, it shoots us straight into a primal, painful swamp of sadness and unworthiness.

We hear a lot about the extremes of jealousy, the leading cause of spousal homicides in the United States. Perpetrated by controlling, possessive people who fly into jealous rages, lacking the support or skill sets to find better ways to deal with their feelings of unworthiness.

But that's not us. We're not stalkers or bad people. Jealousy has a purpose. The entire human race is wired for jealousy as a mechanism for keeping us connected. That's right, jealousy is about survival. It's not a character flaw or something we must pay penance for. Jealousy does not mean we have low self-esteem, are mean spirited, or wish others harm for having what we don't.

Jealousy is what we feel when faced with the threat of not belonging, of disconnection, of being left out, or of having our trust betrayed. It's a warning sign that we've been abandoned or are at eminent risk of losing something or someone we value. Jealousy is born from our deeply primal need to belong.

Exercise: How Do We Reckon with Jealousy?

Spend a few minutes tapping into a current or past situation in which you felt jealous. Sink into it. Ugh. Yes, a toxic swamp of confusing emotions. Consider these positive strategies for managing jealousy successfully:

Breathe into your strong center. Be there.

Then, get into your body. Blow out the strong energy of jealousy through intense full-body movement—a brisk walk, run, big chores, or a tough workout at the gym. Disconnect from your stories about it. Let it flow through.

Affirm: I belong. I belong to myself. I am my whole, true, authentic self.

Consider: What assumptions are you making? Do you have all the facts?

Check your self-judgment. You're not a bad person for feeling jealous!

Claim full responsibility for your painful feelings and let their wisdom guide you to constructive change. Learn to celebrate the successes of your friends as well as your own.

And, suck it up! In the end, life is and always will be unfair. There will always be people who have the goods and the successes we wish we had. Who are better at something, more fortunate, born to more privilege, or are bigger, faster, richer, smarter,

HEAL KARYN SHANKS MD

prettier than we are—always! Why limit yourself? Perhaps there's a bigger, better ship waiting for you right around the corner. Life's unfairness is a simple matter of how we choose to see it (it's a story).

Despair and Hopelessness

It's so easy to sink into despair and hopelessness when we're suffering. Persistent fatigue, pain, and debilitating symptoms that go on and on are the conditions that make us vulnerable to losing hope, especially when we are unsupported in our journey. But as we've discussed and seen, the antidote to despair is hope. Hope is a decision. To allow the future to bring better things. And hope is a practice. It becomes our strength and resilience in the face of despair.

Exercise: How Do We Reckon with Despair and Hopelessness?

As always, first we breathe. We find our strong center. We sit right here in our strong center and breathe.

We get into our bodies. We walk in nature and receive her beauty and energy of the ground, sky, plants, and animals. We hand her our despair and hopelessness. We reach out to our most trusted friends and family, those who can hear us and hold the space (not judge or "fix").

Affirm: Yes. This too shall pass.

Consider: As we breathe into our strong center, we recall that we can do this hard thing whether we believe in it or not. Then, maybe, just maybe, we make the decision to hope. We say "yes" to hope. Whether we believe it or not. Without clinging to a particular outcome, we say "yes." And we persist. And in so doing, we open the gate to our new path, the one we perhaps can't see clearly yet (or at all). We open ourselves to infinite possibilities.

THE POWER OF HOPE

Hope is not just an antidote to despair or our difficult emotions. It's what energizes all our work to claim our truth—to say "yes," to find our strong center, to stand bravely in the face of our uncomfortable emotions. Hope is what keeps us alive and moves us forward.

Hope Is a Decision—My Pain Story

"You *will* get better."

That's what my new rehab doctor said after my first visit, utterly stunning me.

I had yet to hear any such words during my multi-year saga of pain and dysfunction. Not one of the perhaps dozen professionals I had sought help from in the past years had given me any scrap of hope that I might recover.

I had had one complicated injury after the next—all part of a hypermobility syndrome that led to overstretched ligaments all over my body, tendon tears, instability, and intractable pain. A previously healthy, highly active woman who thrived on athletic pursuits, I was suddenly sidelined, barely able to walk, and unable to do what I loved. Heck, I struggled to unload the dishwasher!

I had surgery, invasive procedures, and massive amounts of therapy under my belt. Nothing seemed to put me back together. Even with the support of my heroic woman story, in my pain and rehab story I felt despairing and lost. Hope was a strenuous and lonely exercise that got harder every day.

Until my rehab doc's words. Simple words, but audacious. But just as my son's words had changed my life story, my doctor's words changed my pain story. I *needed* to hear them. For the first time in several years, I felt buoyant with hope. My new story jump-started my journey to full recovery and healing. My new story was hope.

He guided my every move, reminding me at every visit that I was making progress, and he expected success. Painstaking as my recovery was, he held my focus on that positive outcome. He also very gently reminded me that pain is in the brain. I had to work hard on my body. I also had to work on my stories. He nailed that one.

I see many people in my consultation room who, like me, have almost given up hope. I say "almost" because something inspired them to come see me. For some it is one last glimmer of possibility perhaps ignited by a friend's recommendation or something they have read. They may have been sick for a very long time, seen many doctors, and received no sustainable solutions for their problems. They may feel deeply traumatized. They often feel abandoned and alone. The story of hopelessness has added greatly to the burden of their illness. But like all humans, they innately believe that tomorrow will be a better day, so they come.

Having hope is vital for the healing process. Hope is the opening in our thinking that something better is possible, that healing is possible. We may not see it or know what it is, but we believe in the possibilities.

Hope, itself, shifts physiology in many supportive directions. It reduces inflammation, positively modulates the stress response, improves circulation and mood, and inspires creative imagination.

Hope bolsters our sense of commitment and empowerment and prepares and energizes us for the work to come.

The foundation of hope is being present to our true emotions, then finding our strong center to draw from this reservoir of strength to hope. Yes, hope is a decision.

FIND CALM WITHIN THE STORM

Emotions have a way of knocking us off balance. From giddying heights to wallowing lows, we can feel we're losing control, reacting to the storm we're in rather than proactively defining our path. Time to stand still. To find our strong center and stay true to our path. And just as a strong tree can withstand the storm, swaying and rocking while anchored by its roots extending deep within the ground, so too can we ground ourselves to gain the strength of the earth. Beyond metaphor, grounding ourselves is real.

Emotional Grounding—Find Your Strong Center

I am grounded.

I am deeply rooted within the earth.

I am nourished and healed by this beautiful earth.

I release all fear and trust that I am eternally safe.

I am calm and strong in my center.

I am worthy of love and all things beautiful.

Emotional grounding is much the same as electrical grounding, a technique to calm the chaotic, destabilizing, potentially destructive potential of intense emotional energy. Grounding allows us to quickly find our strong center, establish present-moment awareness, and establish a strong, stabilizing foundation with our bodies. Physical contact between our bodies and the earth is helpful here, as it creates a sensory and energetic experience that is calming and strengthening. With grounding we're working directly with the first through third emotional centers, while providing strength and energy for them all.

What Being Ungrounded Feels Like

People who are not grounded feel anxious, disconnected, spacey, and isolated. They have difficulty focusing and connecting to their inner wisdom. They struggle with deciphering internal guidance and making decisions. Ungrounded people may feel "outside" of their bodies, a common experience associated with high anxiety. By connecting the foundational parts of our bodies—feet, legs, hips, pelvis, core, and solar plexus—with the earth, we use these points of contact to move energy through these emotional centers and bolster our embodied presence.

How Grounding Works

The use of focused breath, movement, posture, and sensory contact with the earth supports grounding through:

- electrical energy from the earth into the body (electrons—sources of protective antioxidants and soothing energy);

- sensory stimulation of the body through contact, movement, and posture—hypofrontality (reduces thought interference, see the chapter six section on embodiment science), greater tactile and mental connection to body;

- relaxation (parasympathetic nervous system engagement, see the chapter four section on biological stress); and

- enhanced present-time awareness.

How to Ground Yourself

You can ground yourself quickly and easily by standing or moving while feeling the soles of your feet against the ground. This can be accomplished by going for a walk or run, moving through yoga poses, doing a workout at the gym, moving through chores, or just standing still wherever you're at, fully conscious of the ground beneath you and the sensations in your body.

Become present to the sensations in your feet as they make contact with the ground: as they land, touch the variety of contours and textures of its surface, and move. Feel the strength in your core as you move and hold yourself upright. Feel the stability and strength as the earth holds you. As one foot lands in front of the other, let the earth support you.

As we discussed in chapter six, a simple technique to amplify sensation on the bottoms of the feet is to use a tennis or lacrosse ball. Stand on one foot at a time and gently roll out the entire sole of the opposite foot by rolling it along the ball. Bring your complete awareness into your feet. Breathe into your feet and legs and practice the embodied breathing exercise from chapter six, to enhance full-body awareness. With practice, this meditation becomes second nature and can be accomplished in seconds for quick and efficient grounding in the body.

Use grounding exercises as antidotes to overthinking and anxiety, when you are having difficulty making a decision, or expressing yourself creatively. Just a few breaths and tuning into the sensations in the lower body can revitalize and stabilize you.

When possible, remove yourself from anxious situations that pull you away from your body and present-moment awareness. Take great care when using meditation practices that remove you from the awareness and stabilizing influence of your body, as they can exacerbate anxiety.

And finally, always check in with yourself as you work with *any* practice: Does it feel right for you? Does it feel strengthening? Is there anxiety or discomfort? Does it make you feel worse? Our goal is to seek stability first: to be fully grounded in the body.

CLAIM YOUR EMOTIONAL GENIUS—EIGHT STRATEGIES

You've learned many strategies throughout this book for strengthening yourself in your pursuit of healing. Let's draw from those now, integrating them to help you learn from this powerful source of wisdom. Once again, you're showing up, going slow, and paying attention. You're finding and inhabiting your strong center. You're employing your breath, your present-moment awareness, and being your own compassionate observer. You're claiming your power as the true leader of your own healing.

Claim Your Emotions as Your Inner Wisdom

Your emotions are your soul's gift of knowledge and wisdom to you. No emotion is wasted. They are always pure and true and on your side.

Become Grounded and Embodied

This makes you sturdy as you get close to your emotions. They are physical sensations. The only way to know them in their pure form and observe them directly is to get into the body. Use movement as an antidote to anxiety or emotional intensity that makes you feel muddled.

Let Your Emotions Speak

Resist the temptation to dismiss, judge, or suppress your emotions. Hear them out. Establish a practice of daily reflection about your feelings through writing, meditation, or contemplation. Let your emotions flow. Let them have their voice. You must create space and get quiet to hear them.

Express Gratitude to Your Emotions

Your emotions bring you wisdom. You may not *feel* grateful. That's okay but honor this part of yourself regardless. This practice will shift you out of the limits imposed by stories and restricting mindsets and lets you get right up close to your emotions. By seeing them through a positive lens, the judging stories dissolve, and they seem less scary. Even the anger, grief, fear, and jealousy have something crucial to teach us and will lead us toward healing and wholeness.

Take Charge of Your Emotions

Breathe into them. Observe them. Don't beat them into submission but see them flow from the perspective of the compassionate, neutral observer. Find the discipline to step back from them to give them space to live and breathe. To this end, resist your stories and judgments about them. Let the emotions speak for themselves. Know that your emotions do not own or define you.

Become Discerning about Your Stories

Many of our stories don't ennoble or serve us. Move your body to shake them off and release intensity. Breathe into them. Find the stability and self-awareness to interrupt your stories, no matter how practiced they are. Resist buying into them. Soften. Is there a more ennobling story? If all your emotions are teachers, what are they trying to say? Looking at them through the lens of love or Life School POV, how do they support you?

Recall How the Emotions You Feel May Not Be Your Own

We are attuned to the energy all around us. The more sensitive among us will easily pick up the energy of others. Scrutinize the unexpected anxiety, irritability, or anger: Is it yours? Or someone else's?

Take Solace in the Flow Aspect of Your Emotions

Your emotions will always move along, given the chance. I love to say: "This too shall pass" to reassure myself when in the presence of uncomfortable emotions. It's *always* true.

EMOTIONAL RESCUE 911

There will be difficult, tumultuous emotions. When these emotions crop up, we benefit from the support of the strong center we've protected and nourished so well. We draw on the stabilizing benefits of our grounding practices. We also need emergency tools to pull out when we're challenged—or blindsided—by difficult emotions.

Exercise: Get into Your Body—Find Your Strong Center—Fast!

Breathe deeply. Breathe into your strong center. Find it. This is your anchor.

Breathe into your feet. Feel the sensations of your feet against the ground. Put all your awareness there. Be there. Feel the points of contact between your feet and the ground. Feel the stability and the solace of the earth beneath you.

Move or walk for increased sensation and present-time awareness. Be fully present to your movement. Breathe, move, and be present.

For high anxiety, get on all fours and place your feet and hands firmly on the ground. Become aware of the contact. Breathe into your feet and hands. Lie down on your back with arms and legs spread. Feel this even greater sensation as your body contacts the ground. Breathe in here. Stay present.

Let your emotions flow as you release your mental engagement with them. Keep your attention on the sensations within your body.

Say to yourself, "This too shall pass."

Exercise: Use Affirmations

Have these affirmations at the ready. Write them down and hang them up where you'll see them— use sticky notes!

I am present in my body.

I am present in my feet.

I am safe and secure in my body.

This too shall pass.

Exercise: Soften and Flow

Sometimes we need to soften the harsh edges of our emotions or the tenacious grip they have on us. We must soften our stories about them. Releasing our grip allows them to flow and gives us needed space for perspective.

I soften.

I soften my skin.

I soften my stories.

I soften my judgments.

Gently say these to yourself. Feel the softening and release. Feel the harsh edges of your emotions soften. As you breathe and ground and stay in your strong center, soften. Let those difficult emotions flow. See them flow right out of your body, into the earth. Breathe in light through the top of the head. Breathe out pain, suffering, anger. Soften.

A WORD ABOUT HEALING EMOTIONAL TRAUMA

Our stories can be quite powerful. As we learned in chapter eight, they are designed by our brains to protect us. It is important to honor this and work to safely and effectively release trauma from the body. It's important to acknowledge that the aftermath of trauma—the persistent stories, fear, and anxiety—has a purpose: to keep us alive. But this trauma can be healed. We can find our strength and learn we are safe again. Even the deepest of suffering can be healed and transformed into wisdom.[24]

For those who have experienced deep emotional trauma and find that high anxiety and intense emotions get in the way of your self-practice, work with a psychotherapist trained in mind-body approaches. They can provide intensive support and guidance in this transformative process and help you learn to trust and feel safe in your body again.

---

[24] A superb resource for working with emotional trauma: James S. Gordon, MD. *The Transformation: Discovering Wholeness and Healing After Trauma.* 2019.

LAST THOUGHTS

We are so strong. All we had to do was become aware of our strong center, of our bodies, and of present time. Through this presence we've learned to trust ourselves and trust the wisdom of our feelings. And in the most difficult of times, we stay in the flow. We trust. We feel. We learn. We thrive. We claim our true potential.

Next, we see what is perhaps now self-evident. How this path is our prize. How the presence that leads to our healing and potential reveals the wonder and miraculousness of our lives. How we *rise* to find meaning, purpose, grace, and awe.

Chapter Ten

RISE

Nourish Meaning, Purpose, Grace, and Awe
(Be Present)

Now, we rise.

We rise with each intention, each decision, each step, each small victory, each celebration of ourselves and our commitment to our healing life. Like exquisite punctuation points honoring us. Yes, we're on our true path.

And we rise big. As our self-care opens space, fuels energy, heals, and nudges (or catapults) us into our potential. Because our clarity and practiced attention to ourselves, our bodies, this moment, and the beauty of the world all around us anchors us in our lives.

This presence is our ultimate healing. And this presence reveals the path as well as the prize—the meaning, purpose, grace, and awe of our entire lives.

MY STORY OF PRESENCE

Sometime in my late thirties it hit me in a serious way: that this whole gig of life, when it all gets boiled down, is really all about being Present. I use a capitol P because it was a big idea and a powerful revelation.

I was driving along on the country road that leads me from home to work, mind wandering as it always does, taking in the beauty of the sunlit countryside, the soft rolling hills, the prairie grasses and the cows. It was early on a summer morning, the sunflowers radiant beneath the rising sun, swaying along the side of the road. As I drove around the curve, observing the old red barn I admired every day, it suddenly came to me—just a thought emerging from the background of many meandering thoughts. It was subtle but distinctly recognizable as something I had better pay attention to. It was just a moment, the beginning of one of those big insights we are graced with sometimes, that catapult us out of our ordinary lives and change everything.

A short time before that day, I'd heard an interview with Houston Smith, the venerable religious scholar, in which he stated that he awakened every single morning greeting the new day with excitement and anticipation. Listening to his words I found myself utterly confused. And jealous. And pissed! I'd been an avid journaler for years, had recently been working with positive affirmations, a gratitude practice, and regular meditation. I was attempting to create new positive neural networks in my brain to shift toward deeper happiness and out of anxiety and overwhelm. But I wasn't there yet, and those first moments of conscious awareness after waking up were always the hardest. I'd worked hard and still wasn't really sure I was ever going to get there. And there was Houston just casually throwing it out there, how grateful and happy he was from the moment he woke up. How could that be? Life was so damned hard! How could he conceivably feel that way? What did he know?

But as I considered Houston's words and my strong response to them, I decided he might have something important to teach me. I began to work with new affirmations every morning: *I am grateful for this new day, it's a beautiful new day, good things are happening today.* No matter how tired, overwhelmed, crabby, or disbelieving I felt on any given day, with the very first break of consciousness, I got to work on feeling better, saying those affirmations.

It was awkward at first because that's not how I actually *felt* during those first flickers of consciousness, especially on work mornings, right on the painful heels of my alarm rousing me from deep sleep. But I wanted those new neural networks like Houston's. So, I kept at it. I started with my new affirmations, then dumped my frustration, stress, and worry into my journal. With my more spacious mind, I expanded on the affirmations by exploring positive solutions to my daily problems. Eventually I didn't have to think about it so hard. I could utter, "It's a beautiful day" as soon as I was awake. Quite miraculously, I felt better in general, and I *did* feel grateful for the new day. I was more optimistic and light hearted. Even those busy mornings of juggling work, kids, and chores became lighter.

In those days I was also letting go to create more space for myself in my life, sleeping more, making key changes in how I ate, and finding more time to move and exercise. I believe all this, with my newfound presence, converged to make me open, attentive, and ready for my big insight on that quiet country road.

In that moment I realized that all my years of effort and hard work to develop myself as a mom, a physician, and a person had involved a forward progression through accumulation, layering on all the qualifications, attributes, and skills that I felt made me more worthy. All my years of learning, of becoming more formally educated, of acquiring new skills and ways of thinking—which I thought would add up to some cumulative score of how successful and valuable I was in this life— turned out not to be the basis of my success and worth at all. I had missed the entire point of what it means to be a successful human being. It's not about *what* we are or *what* we achieve. It's not a *what* at all. It's an *is*. It's about just *being*. Being totally, openly, fully... us. Present.

I felt relieved. I felt released from pursuing a goal that could never be achieved, the burden of a lifetime of tyranny to be something better than I was. I am the product of a culture that defines our worthiness by action and accomplishment. We are taught we must *earn* our status. We must work hard, go to school, climb the ladder, claw our way up the next higher mountain. It's all about effort and leaning in. What gets left out of our training is the simple fact that we are inherently worthy just as we are. That we are miracles just for being. That we are blessings to this world by virtue of being ourselves without having to prove it. I had spent a lifetime working hard to achieve the success I already had. I just didn't know it. Or maybe I had forgotten. That day on the country road, I woke up.

For me it was a revelation that it's all about *being*: about *successfully being* rather than being successful. It's not all about acquisition and rewards. Acquiring knowledge and skill is important, benefiting me and those I serve in many profound ways. But, in the end, they are tools for me to use. They don't make me a more successful person. My success is already here. It's ordained. My charge is to see it. To know it. To claim it. And when I do, then I'm free. Free to use the tools for others. Free to grow. Free to experience the moment. Free to do whatever I want, because I'm no longer limited by the false notion that I have to prove myself. I can grow. I can achieve my untapped potential simply because that's who I am.

I arrived at work that day feeling like a new person. But I wasn't really new. I'd had a life-changing, life-affirming revelation, but my work had just begun. It would take years for that revelation to translate into new ways of living and thinking about myself, to replace the old ways, and I am still very much a work in progress. My work has not been to add layers, but to peel them away. To become more aware, tuned in, and Present to it all—to me, to the people and things around me, to life.

The work of becoming more Present has revealed to me the greatest gifts of this life. When we're Present, the meaningful parts of our lives are illuminated and the unneeded parts are shed.

HOW WE RISE—MEANING, PURPOSE, GRACE, AND AWE

The fruits of all our work to heal are in how we move closer to our potential—how we rise.

Meaning and Purpose

We all look for the meaning and purpose of our lives. Meaning is what inspires us. And purpose is how we take that inspiration into our lives, how we leave our personal touch on our world. When we're present, the meaning is clearer—we feel it, we can access it—and our purpose unfolds organically as we live through that meaning. And it's way less complicated than we make it sometimes.

Not clinging to the past or worrying about the future frees up our awareness and appreciation for what is. It's all pretty simple. Be a good person. Love a lot. Spread your light. It's not complicated or sophisticated. It's not about winning, getting straight As, or being the best. It's not about the great career or extraordinary accomplishments, unless you bring your full presence and shine your light through them.

At first glance my grandmother Harriet, an elementary school teacher in a small town in Illinois, would seem to have little in common with President Barack Obama. Yet they both used their positions to share their Presence and spread their light. Through her gentle voice and her supporting hand on a shoulder, my grandmother was present to her sacred work in those young lives, and so inspired generations of schoolchildren. Many came back as adults to thank her and share memories. President Obama may have had the power of the presidency behind him, but it was his listening, his caring, his Presence that captivated people around the globe. Both Harriet and Barak are examples of highly successful people. Not because of their jobs, but because of the Presence and light they brought to their work—their meaning and purpose shined through their jobs.

Grace

Grace is the energy of possibility and potential. Grace is the smooth intuitive connection between movements. Grace is the seamless flow from thought to thought to new ideas. Grace is the firm but gentle hand on our shoulder that both supports us and assures that we're on the right track.

Grace, like all energy of the world, is there for us. It flows in when we welcome it. When we soften. When we let go of excessive effort or rigid expectations. When we let go of the distractions and suffering that yank us out of present time.

We're approached by grace when we take pause, breathe, pay attention, allow for the unexpected, and believe in the infinite possibilities of our lives. While grace is always there and its work unbidden, it is, paradoxically, also a decision we choose to make.

Grace can come as an answer. A message. Guidance. Synchronicity. "By grace," we say. I found an answer by grace. I was led to exactly what I needed by grace. I met you by grace. My failure transformed into magnificence by grace. It is the divine element of our world, playing its dutiful role in our lives at all times. It supports and guides us always and continues to be there even when we forget, worry, conjure up obstructive stories, and let fear about tomorrow take hold of us.

When we're present, the grace flows in—we see the grace that was always there.

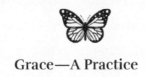

Grace—A Practice

Pause here. Breathe deeply.

Feel your Presence.

Now say, "thank you," opening yourself to grace.

Grace is all around us. We manifest it instantly through our gratitude for what we have and who we are right now. You see, gratitude opens the channel for grace to flow into us. It's the divinity in our present-moment awareness that our wide-open eyes and hearts can take in and experience. The grace was always there. We found it when we learned to connect to our strong center. Oh, my gosh, grace is within us.

Awe

"The great lesson from the true mystics is that the sacred is in the ordinary, that it is to be found in one's daily life, in one's neighbors, friends, and family, and in one's backyard."

—*Abraham H. Maslow, Religions, Values, and Peak-Experiences*

We all know awe from those amazing soul-smacking experiences that we don't expect: the incredible sunsets, enormous rainbows, powerful storms, expressions of big love, and moments of drop-to-our-knees grace. This is the awe that pulls us out of our ordinary everyday experiences to heighten our senses and transform us forever.

Though we may not recognize it as such at the time, awe can also come to us as the tragedies, colossal disappointments, and failures. The common factor in all these experiences is how they expand us, remove us from ordinary space and time, and create our sense of the world as much larger than ourselves.

Abraham Maslow spoke of awe as those *peak-experiences* that are "rare, exciting, oceanic, deeply moving, exhilarating, elevating experiences that generate an advanced form of perceiving reality, and are even mystical and magical in their effect upon the [person]." He considered these states of mind to be the mark of the fully actualized human and, in fact, the goal of people desiring to become more fully awake, alive, and present.

Albert Einstein, a seeker and searcher, realized how central awe was to his work and to the beauty of the human experience. In reflecting on it he said, "The most beautiful thing we can experience is the mysterious. It is the source of all true art and science. He to whom the emotion is a stranger, who can no longer pause to wonder and stand wrapped in awe is as good as dead—for their eyes are closed."

Awe is a central part of being human. We're *wired* for awe. Experiences of awe create positive changes in physiology with reduced markers of inflammation and stress. Scientific observation of awe reveals that we become more expansive and creative, experience a greater sense of connection with one another, an elevated sense of purpose about our lives, and deeper gratitude when in the face of awe-inspiring experiences. Those extraordinary expansions of consciousness teach and strengthen us. From the earthshaking events to the small miracles, the elements of awe are all there, surrounding us, positioned to launch us toward better health, deeper connections, and our higher selves.

Awe can stimulate change. The events of 9/11 catapulted us all into a sense of communal strength and purpose like no other time in our recent history. I leaped from one career to another that year, inspired by the sense of there being no time to waste, and that I must step up to my true purpose. I left my job with a hospital to open my own practice founded on the principles of Functional Medicine and body-mind healing.

Awe can create connection. Witnessing the births of our children opens us to one of our lives' greatest miracles, preparing us for the work and transformation yet to come. I was flung into unimagined depths of concern for another's survival and wellbeing, of true sacrifice, and of profound connection unlike any I had experienced before.

Awe can open our eyes to the moment. On vacation, my husband and I drove right through an enormous double rainbow in Hawaii. We could see both ends of the massive arch as it was suspended right over us. I was slack-jawed the entire time (the facial expression of awe), my eyes and smile big. We were suspended in that moment, beneath the double rainbow, which had graced our path.

Awe is the experience of grace in action. It's the connection we feel to our world when we pay attention. Often, we are limited to experiencing awe only when it spectacularly crosses our path. But we can also experience awe daily, in our ordinary lives, when our eyes are wide open and we are awake and aware, by paying closer attention to what's going on—*really going on*—around us. We connect with the miracles and magic of life that constantly surrounds us. We don't have to wait for the cataclysmic and catastrophic events of our lives to force us into the present moment. It doesn't have to be the double rainbows.

PRESENCE—THE PATH IS THE PRIZE

Meaning, purpose, grace, and awe are the beauty of our lives. Each begets and supports the other. But the gateway to them all—revealing the path as well as the prize—is Presence.

I had *eight* domains for the first version of this book, each representing the essential elements and practices that lead us to our destination. Then I realized that our destination is also our path there. Reverent self-care leads to Presence, and Presence supports our work. Presence is the central thread of all the domains of healing—of all our lives. Our success is in the showing up, going slow, and paying attention that allows us to access our healing.

Presence is the way. Presence is also our reward.

We know by now that Presence is not passive. Presence isn't about sitting still and waiting. Or hoping things will work out well. Presence is the greatest challenge of our lives. It's hard, but it rewards us. It takes courage, but it expands us. It leads us along our healing path. It's our go-to tool for slowing down and letting go of toxins, irritants, distractions, and negative energy. It allows us to love and connect deeply to others. It shows us our strong center and strengthens us in the face of life's challenges. It helps us to rest, sleep, and restore. Then to move with strength and stability. It guides us as we make food choices that nourish us and fuel our energy. And it holds the space for navigating our stories and realizing the infinite potential of our lives. Presence helps us hold on as we're brave to feel, trusting the inner genius of our emotions.

Presence is our tool. Presence is our path. And Presence is our prize. It's how we *rise*.

LAST THOUGHTS

Throughout this book we've explored the domains of healing and considered ways to improve our lives. We've considered our starting points, our paths, and our desired destinations. I truly hope you're living better and feeling better than you did when you started this book. But this process takes time. It's far easier to read about something you desire than to actually do it and keep going.

As we strive for change and healing, what do we do with the setbacks and disappointments—the failures—that are the inevitable part of the progress forward? We breathe. We find our center. We stay present. We turn the page.

Chapter Eleven

PARTING WORDS: BOW TO FAILURE

Finally, we must fail. Failure is our finest, wisest, most spectacular teacher. No other source of guidance is as attuned to our every thought and action. Without her we would have no path at all. No true path. No path worth taking.

Failure puts on the brakes when we need them. Kicks us in the butt when we're slacking. And gets our attention when we journey in the wrong direction.

We are graced with our failures, but mistake and malign them as our disappointments, the cause of our suffering and unrealized expectations. We use our setbacks as our excuse to avoid change, the very change we need to unleash our true potential.

THE CONUNDRUM OF THINGS NOT WORKING OUT

It starts like this, doesn't it? We feel the terrible sting of disappointment because things are not turning out as we hoped. Our expectations are not met. A door slams in our face and we feel devastated. Or, in spite of working really, really hard, our savvy plan seems to go nowhere.

Then what?

You know, by now, where I'm going here, right?

Yep, we make up a story. Something like this: "I failed." Or, "I *am* a failure." Or, "*they* failed me." Or, "I suck at this. " Or, "there's no hope for me."

Somehow, we got it all wrong. Somewhere along the line we decided that when things don't work out it says something very personal and very terrible about us or someone else.

What's with that? Sounds ridiculous when we stop and think about it, doesn't it? But we all do it. We all make up disparaging stories about these pivotal moments of change that could be moments of genius if we'd let them. Let's take a closer look.

MY STORY OF FAILURE

My whole practice of medicine—my identity as a physician, my philosophy of what constitutes healing, and my approach to my clients—has been built on a series of failures.

I tried to become an academic physician after four years of medical school and my three-year residency in internal medicine. You know, ivory towers and the "truth." I wanted to be part of that. In the center of it all. Where innovation and great wisdom came to bear. I knew I had the intelligence, the drive, and the ability to succeed. I spoke to my department chair, and he enthusiastically agreed to take me on as faculty as soon as I finished my residency. But there was a problem. You see, I was expecting my first child at the end of my residency and I was passionate about spending as much time with my new baby as possible. I told my chair this, and he initially agreed that I could work part-time.

But then, when my new son was just a couple months old and before I actually had to start work, my chair changed his mind. "*Professional* physicians work full time," he told me. I was stunned. It was certainly his prerogative to run his department as he saw fit, and back in the early 1990s, physicians simply didn't work part-time. I knew this. But I was determined to be my child's primary care provider. I could not imagine handing him over to a fulltime nanny or daycare center. That's what all the other professional moms I knew did to have both careers and children, but I could not do it. It's not that what other moms did was wrong, it just wasn't for me.

I loved my work and was passionate about becoming a great doctor and building a medical practice. I wanted both, on my terms. But my plans hit a brick wall. In my desire to be the kind of mom I wanted to be, I had failed as an academic physician. My chair's words reverberated inside me: *You're not a professional physician if you work-part time.* I doubted myself. Was I a wimp? I felt deflated. Kicked out of the kingdom. Ostracized.

Demoted. And lost. I felt lost. Couldn't I be a good mom on the terms that felt right to me as well as an excellent physician?

I knew in my core that my child and my goals for myself as a parent must come first. Not only that but I knew (I knew!) that it would, in fact, make me a better doctor to live a more balanced life than what I observed in many of my mentors and colleagues. Eighty-to ninety-hour work weeks and being on-call overnight and on weekends were standard—crazy, but standard. I knew I wasn't alone in my thinking, but I was certainly alone in my actions: turning down an academic position because the imbalance of long work hours and precious time with my new son. I knew there was a better way for me. I *knew* this.

So, I had to shift directions and find my own path. I was passionately in love with my new son. I let him inspire my new direction. I took a temporary part-time position at an outlying family practice clinic in a rural area and eventually joined an internal medicine group, then was hired by a hospital to launch their new integrative medicine program. I worked part-time in all these jobs and managed to balance family and my career. Eventually I ended up where I am now, founder and director of my own unique and successful practice that uses these same core values of whole-person body-mind-life balance to address needs of clients with chronic complex illness.

In retrospect I'm thankful that I was so stubborn and resolute. I stayed my course in spite of my deep feelings that I had failed. Though the experience was painful, I knew, without a moment of doubt or hesitation, that I had made the correct choice. I would not know for many years to come that the choice was a pivotal moment for me as a doctor and a healer.

My choice to stick to my guns about working part-time to create more room for motherhood and a balanced life, placed me squarely on a path of personal discovery and evolution that would lead me to a richer understanding of human beings and what constitutes healing, and a better understanding of my true role as a physician—as partner, mentor, and guide. I was led to change my understanding of what the best medicine *is*, and to become one of the pioneers of a revolutionary sea change in medicine throughout our country and around the world. I am proud of that. In retrospect, I am so relieved that the door to academic medicine closed on me at that critical juncture of my life.

This is just one example of how the most profound, deep, and meaningful lessons of my life have come from my "failures." I had to learn that it's not personal. And it's not about screwing up. There are reasons that things don't always turn out the way we plan.

DECONSTRUCTING FAILURE

Failure is, in essence, when things don't go as planned. When this happens, one of three things is usually true.

- There is something we need to learn.

- There is something else we need to do first.

- What we planned is just not meant to be.

Notice how I list those three reasons for failure with no emotion attached to them. We need to learn something; we need to do something first; or it's not meant to be. Period.

None of them say we're bad people. None of them say we're weak. None of them say anything at all about us. Each is a specific instruction, a direction, a roadmap for what to do next.

My husband failed in his first major research grant proposal because he needed to learn how to write an effective proposal. My son failed in writing his first machine-learning algorithm in graduate school because he needed to preprocess his data first. I failed in my first medical path because I needed to go in a different direction. None of these "failures" were about us as people. Just lessons to be learned. Not end points. We've all moved on. My husband has now received numerous grants. My son is creating new computer algorithms daily, and my medical path—well, it's been mind-blowingly transformational!

The only possible failure is in giving up.

In retrospect, I see that if I hadn't failed at key points in my life, I wouldn't be who I am or have what I have. Failure has saved my butt. And all the rejections, abandonments, injuries, and setbacks were my teachers, without which I would not be who I am today. All Life School. All those "failures" morphed into profound lessons and understanding and have led to deeper freedom and happiness. And all of them have taught me that failure is just a matter of perception. They're just stories. That's right. In the end, failure is just a story.

Failure Is a Story

"There is only one reason that a company fails. When the entrepreneur gives up. That's it. Period. No other reason."

—Adeo Ressi, *The Founder Institute*

We've established that failure is not about our personal shortcomings or anything we've done wrong.

Failure, plain and simple, is Life School.

However, as a culture we've added negative connotations—stories—to the word. Like stress, failure is neither good nor bad, it describes a situation that is value neutral.

These stories we tell about failure can be powerful.

Every client I see brings a story of failure. Their stories often involve many years of searching for answers and seeing many doctors in various institutions, all to no avail. Maybe they have gone through repeated attempts at weight loss, using a variety of popular regimens without success or diets that were not sustainable. Or failed attempts to take on important new lifestyle practices because the change required losing something they couldn't let go of. Everyone has these stories. And they are all valuable. They all have meaning. They all contain key bits of data and should be used to discover the truth.

But we need to understand—*really* understand—that the emotions we attach to our "failures" are just stories. They are not the truth. And as we've seen, our stories are inspired by the assumptions and fears that delude us into seeing our circumstances in particular ways. Often ways that demean and disempower us.

Yes, life brings us deep disappointments and sadness. And we must honor and grieve our losses. Our failed food plans and exercise goals are no exception.

But we have to see that each of these situations presents us with opportunities to decide: Do we judge and condemn ourselves for not meeting our expectations? Or do we regroup, reassess, get smarter, more supported, and start again?

When we can arrive at this understanding, the shame and suffering for our disappointments and upended plans is transformed. Give your suffering its due, then forgive yourself, and make the decision to move on.

Failure Is Not Personal

When we understand that our failures are not personal, we can see them in a whole new light.

All our actions and decisions are experiments that we direct.

And as experiments, the outcomes will not always be what we expect.

That's life, and we must be patient with its uncertainty. Unexpected outcomes and being pushed in new directions may frustrate us, disappoint us, get in the way of our plans, and greatly inconvenience us, but they are quite possibly taking us to a better place. When we see this, we can exercise a deeper level of responsibility for our actions and their outcomes and what they mean.

I cannot stress enough that my own life has been a series of miracles that would have never happened if I had resisted those opportunities, ignored them, or persisted in my old ways. We fail. We must fail. And we must ask: Is there something else I must learn? Is there something else I need to do first? Do I need to try a different path? Don't get stuck in your stories. Move on.

Failure Makes Us More Successful Human Beings

"Fail, fail again, fail better."

—*Pema Chödrön*

We fail. We *must* fail.

It's key to understand that while a single failure may seem like a big thing in the moment, it's just a moment. I don't mean to dismiss it. But in this whole book we're talking about something much bigger than a moment—we're talking about our lives. And from that perspective, we should welcome failure with open arms.

Our failures, disappointments, and challenges build character. Didn't our parents tell us that? They make us stronger if we don't give up. They foster resilience and creativity. They're the challenge that creates our strong center. When what we want comes easily, great! But, so what? We may quickly and easily get what we want. But the easiest way is not necessarily the most fruitful or rewarding way.

Having to struggle or try again is not a sign that we have failed as human beings or that the gods aren't smiling on us. It's how we function. It's the logical expression of how we learn through taking action. Remember our discussion about stress? Stress and failure go hand in hand. In the same way that a body without stress can't respond to stress with growth and development and success, a person without failure will never be given the opportunities to develop to their highest potential.

The Law of Attraction is Misleading

I think the popular understanding of the law of attraction oversimplifies what it takes to create the life we want. It teases us with the illusion that we can control every outcome if we just think and feel correctly.

This way of thinking leads us to judge ourselves when we run into difficulty. It *shames* us for failing.

The law of attraction inspires tools to help us change in positive directions, to harness the energy of neuroplasticity and epigenetics. But it is not a primary truth. The things that happen to us aren't the result of simple cause and effect: think it, believe it, chant it, and it will come. No. We're way more nuanced and complex than that. And thank God.

The path to getting what we want contains twists and turns that we can't anticipate, don't expect, and require us to actively respond to outcomes. They may be frustrating. We may become disenchanted or discouraged or think it's our fault. But these experiences of "failure" may contain those necessary elements that carve us into our greater selves in ways that we could never plan or predict on our own. They are the mysterious and miraculous parts of our journey that no planning could ever account for.

Yes, we *must* fail. If we allow it, failure is the crucible that leads to something new, something better, something even more successful.

The "Three Tack Rule"

> *"This food plan isn't working for me."*
>
> *"This treatment has done absolutely nothing."*
>
> *"I thought I'd be feeling better by now. This is a failure."*

Healing can be so hard. And take so long. What if you're working hard and not feeling any better?

This happens. A lot. And it's important to not mistake "failure" for something not working out. You're going to find that many of the things you try in order to heal don't work for you. That may not mean they aren't good for you.

It may mean there's more to do.

One of my Functional Medicine mentors, Dr. Sidney Baker, speaks of what he calls "the three tack rule."

It goes like this: If you sit on three tacks, they hurt like hell and no amount of symptomatic treatment will make it feel better.

If you take one tack away, or better yet two, you've taken care of two-thirds of the problem. That's huge! But you still hurt like hell. You may not even recognize how much you've accomplished.

It's only when you remove that third remaining tack that the pain goes away.

Still, removal of each successive tack was critical to resolving the whole problem at the root cause level.

We're Not Failures, We're Complicated!

We often have to address many aspects of a complex problem before our suffering is relieved. This doesn't mean that each step in the process isn't important. It doesn't mean we've failed. It just means that we are complex. We have to tend to the whole of the problem to make real progress.

If you and your health team believe that what you are doing is important to your overall health and healing, hang in there. There is more to do before there is enough recovery for you to actually feel better. Keep the faith.

Your "Failure" is Showing You a Better Path

There are also times when the treatment plan is wrong for you. It is often impossible to know this until you embark on the journey and make a commitment to a particular path. But that still isn't failure. It's learning what you need to know—from what *didn't* work—to lead you toward a better path for you.

How Do We Manage These "Failures?"

Remain aware of your body and your feelings. Check in with your team. Work together toward a meaningful change in direction and recommit.

As you keep the faith, ask yourself: Is there something else I need to learn? Is there something else I need to do first? Am I on the right path?

Hope Neutralizes the Sting of Failure

Dealing with the frustration of failure can be tough. I know this so well.

But we have the most powerful tool in our arsenal to deal with it: hope.

You, right now, wherever you are on your journey, can hope. Whether you actually feel it or not, you have it—you're still with us at the end of this book, yes? What's kept you here? Hope. It's powerful medicine.

Hope is what energizes our way forward. It's what pulls us out of the pain of disappointment, disempowerment, and despair. It reminds us failure is not forever.

And hope is in us—it's part of us.

Hope is the decision that we make to believe that things can be better, and it is the tool we use to make them better, energizing what we do next. And like everything else we have discussed in this book hope is a practice.

Hope is the decision—it's when we say "yes."

Grit Energizes Hope

First we hope, but how do we create real world solutions?

Grit comes next. It's how we take that next step in total faith, not seeing the way forward. It's the toughness that helps us to persevere when things are really hard. It's how we embrace hope when we hurt like hell. How we create new stories that nourish us and help us to rise up out of our current circumstances to aspire to something new and better.

Grit is hope in action. It takes courage. It's our decision to go forward squarely into the face of the unknown, ignoring the stories of possible misfortune, keeping a laser-sharp focus on our desires. Grit is how we embrace hope, knowing that our current perceptions, experiences, and feelings do not fully define who we are or the trajectory of our lives. As humans we get to be much bigger than that. The courageous journey we choose for ourselves is fortifying. It builds resilience. And from time to time we get to experience the thrill and miracle of success. We get to be reborn. We always move toward our full potential.

HEAL: A LIFELONG COMMITMENT TO ENLIGHTENED FAILURE

"People who wade into the discomfort and vulnerability and tell the truth about their stories are the real badasses."

—*Brené Brown, Rising Strong*

A client recently told me: "Self-care is not for sissies." So true. And yet, while it can be difficult, there is no higher calling than what we do for ourselves. It is our greatest legacy and our gift to this world.

I will close with a manifesto to *us*, to creating our best selves through the risky business of enlightened failure: how to transform our usual self-judging thinking about failure as a character flaw to failure as beauty and information, rich with insights about who we are and what we need to serve and guide us at every step. No longer are our missteps and disappointments evidence of our weakness. They are our intuitive guidance showing us a better way.

So, listen up. Pay attention to yourself. Failure is inevitable. And there is no finer teacher to help us navigate the journey of our lives and, ultimately, our healing.

We *Must* Fail

"The most promising words ever written on the map of human knowledge are terra incognita—unknown territory."

—Daniel J. Boorstein, *The Discoverers*

Here's my final and most important piece of advice: Screw up, fall down, mess up.

That's the only way you'll ever be able to prove to yourself that you risked trying. Every moment of every day, you are walking into the unknown. As you embark on your healing journey, you can have no idea of the exact path you will follow. There *will* be change. How the change occurs will be uncertain. There are risks: you might be wrong, you might be right, you might have to try really hard, you might have to ask for help (it's not that bad!), you may get in over your head, and you will inevitably have to learn new things about yourself and what you are made of.

It all takes great courage. And, inevitably, you will fail.

And when you do fail, you must be tender with yourself as life offers up its most precious lessons to you in this way. The lessons that you give birth to yourself out of your effort, determination, and creativity. Your failures are the guideposts, the intuitive guidance, the divine intervention that redirect you down a new and unexpected path, the path that is better for you at this time or that closes doors to old ways that no longer serve you. We must learn to say "thank you" instead of hanging our heads.

Final Exercise: Failure Mining

Think about a spectacular failure. How do you feel about it now? Still feel that sting of shame, guilt, or sheepishness? Write this story down.

Now, tell a different story. A new, shiny, and ennobling story.

What did you learn from your brush with failure? How did it shed light on a situation that no longer worked for you? In spite of your dashed hopes or unrealized expectations, did in move you in a new and better direction?

If you still have not recovered from that failure, I want you to reframe it now. Explore it from the Life School POV and see it through the lens of love. Assume it happened to save you. To steer you in a better direction. To help you create a better life. Write that story in as much beautiful detail as you can. Then live that story—your true story.

Stand Proudly

On April 23, 1910 in Paris, France, Theodore Roosevelt delivered one of the most widely quoted speeches of his career entitled, "Citizenship in a Republic." He railed against a trend of cynics who looked down at people who were trying to make the world a better place. Considering what you're trying to accomplish in your life by reading this book, in dealing with the inevitable setbacks, in dealing with the people around you who may not be as supportive as you'd like, I think Roosevelt's words apply. How we take care of ourselves is how we take care of our world. This precious gift of life—ours, of those around us, of our planet—is in our care. Making ourselves better will make the world better. Be strong. Stay centered. And when you fall, stand proudly up, brush yourself off, think of this quote, and smile.

"It is not the critic who counts; not the man who points out how the strong man stumbles, or where the doer of deeds could have done them better. The credit belongs to the man who is actually in the arena, whose face is marred by dust and sweat and blood; who strives valiantly; who errs, who comes short again and again, because there is no effort without error and shortcoming; but who does actually strive to do the deeds; who knows great enthusiasm, the great devotions; who spends himself in a worthy cause; who at the best knows in the end the triumph of high achievement and who at the worst, if he fails, at least fails while daring greatly, so that his place shall never be with those cold timid souls who neither know victory nor defeat."

HEAL

Now go celebrate you. Celebrate your commitment to your healing life. To your potential. Celebrate each and every step, no matter how small or humble, made in the spirit of your growth and healing. Know that I am with you—we're all with you—as we take this journey together. The human journey. The journey of discovery, of enlightened failure, of Presence. It is the journey toward the energy and potential we all seek. To heal ourselves, our lives, our world. I bow to you all.

ACKNOWLEDGEMENTS

I lay this book at the feet of my true teachers and companions in this healing life—my clients. People from all walks of life who've sat across from me, trusting me with their stories, bravely stepping up to the call of their illnesses, and helping teach me everything I know about the miracle of life and healing. I can't thank you enough. This book is for you and only possible because of you.

I am grateful to the Institute for Functional Medicine for reintroducing me to the foundational principles of human biological function (that got scattered in the maze of conventional medical training and practice) so I could integrate them with the art of caring for human beings in deep and meaningful ways: through rigorous attention to individuals' life stories, their unique systems biology (with no detail left out), and personal aspirations for healing—to unlock the healing power within them. Thank you for teaching me the tools that keep the complex simple and the chaos organized. And, most importantly, for reigniting my passion for medicine.

Thank you to the skilled and caring healers who showed up in my own life at just the right times, listened carefully to my own story, then walked the path of my healing life with me. Your insights, guidance, encouragement, and love have healed me. You know who you are.

The journey of book writing became way less lonely with the help and companionship of friends, co-writers, readers, and editors. Betsy Rippentrop was there from the very first bubble chart I created to trace the flow of my initial ideas for this book—it may have contained every thought I'd ever had! Your encouragement and celebration of those early steps were priceless. Linda Sivertsen and co-participants at the Carmel writer's retreat showed me the strengths of the book and helped me believe I could produce something of value. Many friends and colleagues read the book in whole (you are true badasses!) or in parts, giving me invaluable feedback that made this book so much better. My editors at kn literary agency knocked it out of the park with each round of editing. You truly taught me how to write. And special thanks to Robin Deutschendorf, my web designer, but so much more. You get me, my story, my medicine, my message, this book. I only have to ask for what I need with about two sentences and you come back with something that blows me away. Thank you for taking such a deep dive into this book's content, creating its beautiful graphics, a gorgeous book cover, insightful messaging to get the word out, and walking me through the steps of book design, formatting, and publishing.

Thank you to my friends and colleagues at the Center for Medicine and Healing Arts. You all do beautiful work and I trust you with each and every one of our precious clients. Shannan Cassidy, my good friend and assistant in all things, I am grateful our clients are in such capable and caring hands from the very first point of contact. Your support helps me to breathe and know it's all okay.

And finally, I am so grateful for my family. From letting me claim our unused dining room for my own writing space over five years ago, tolerating my decreased attention to household tasks, to your unfailing belief in me. Mostly thank you for being my family: the beautiful container of love, adventure, and belonging that makes my life complete. This book gave me a new direction when Sean and Aidan launched themselves into the world. You guys are amazing. Rosie, Nutmeg, and Jasper, your soft fuzziness and playfulness have kept me grounded. And Brian, you read every word of this book many times, offering insights and ideas that breathed greater depth, breadth, and truth to it, in spite of being in the most challenging time of your life. There really aren't words. But you'd push me to find them, wouldn't you? Thanks. And I love you.

APPENDIX A

DEPRIVATION: HOW TO COPE

Changing how we eat—or changing *anything*—can seem daunting, but it's doable when we get organized and break it up into manageable steps.

The hardest part for most of us is dealing with deprivation. We are attached to our food, our ways, our habits even if they hurt us.

I once challenged myself to giving up *all* sugar. I was already close, but I needed to kick my chocolate chip habit—yikes. My guilty pleasure, that got me through the "witching hour," the first few moments of walking into my house after a long day at work, shaking off the intensity of the day, and stepping into the intensity of my household—dogs needing to be greeted, then walked and fed, dinner to get ready, expectations (real or imagined) of my family to tend to. I sought refuge in that bag of Ghirardelli semi-sweet chocolate chips that always, *always* sat on my pantry shelf. Its sole purpose to provide me with the solace and energy I needed to transition from the frying pan into the fire.

So, I gave them up. And my world turned upside down. Literally. What the hell?

Enter one of my yoga teachers with a simple meditation to manage the deprivation of letting go. She called it, "seeding the gap." The gap where we feel left hanging, abandoned, desperate by our precious sacrifice. She taught me to "seed" that gap with a new intention. It goes like this:

Create the intention to make that small change. Step up into action. Feel the pain, the loss, the *deprivation* created by that small sacrifice, and the gap it creates in your experience. Then seed it with something new. An intention. A blessing. A gratitude. Repurpose the deprivation—deploy the energy of it to support your aspirations for yourselves. For me it was, "Thank you, Universe, for supporting my best health and wellbeing." "Thank you for my perfect health." "Thank you for my highest, wisest self."

How to Seed the Gap of Your Own Sacrifice

- List five reasons why you want to create change (in whatever arena of your life this may be—how you eat, sleep, move, think, or otherwise take care of yourself). What about you or your life do you want to change?

- Make a declarative statement—your *decision*—about your desired change (remember: keep the statement positive and present tense):

- Where do you want to start? List the three actions you can take today to energize your decision to change:

- Anticipate the deprivation you may (and probably will) experience as you implement your changes. How will you "seed the gap?"

APPENDIX B

THE HEAL EXERCISES, PRACTICES, AND PERMISSION SLIPS

REFERENCES AND FURTHER READING

CHAPTER ONE

What is Functional Medicine: ifm.org/functional-medicine/.

Karyn Shanks. "What is Functional Medicine?" 2017: karynshanksmd.com/what-is-functional-medicine/

Norman Doidge, MD. *The Brain That Changes Itself.* 2007.

Kenneth R. Pelletier. *Change Your Genes, Change Your Life: Creating Optimal Health with the New Science of Epigenetics.* 2018.

CHAPTER TWO

Brené Brown. *Braving the Wilderness: The Quest for True Belonging and the Courage to Stand Alone.* 2017.

Eyal Ophir, et al. "Cognitive Control in Media Multitaskers." *PNAS* September 15, 2009 106(37): 15583–15587: doi.org/10.1073/pnas.0903620106.

Edita Poljac, et al. "New Perspectives on Human Multitasking." *Psychological Research.* January 2018, Volume 82, Issue 1, pp 1–3: link.springer.com/article/10.1007/s00426-018-0970-2. Editorial with comprehensive list of recent research addressing the problems associated with multitasking by humans.

Karyn Shanks, MD. "Simplicity: The Fine Art of Doing Just One Thing." 2017: karynshanksmd.com/2017/04/05/simplicity-the-fine-art-of-doing-just-one-thing/.

American Psychological Association. "Driven to Distraction: Driving and Cell Phones Don't Mix." 2006: apa.org/research/action/drive.aspx.

The National Safety Council. "Distracted Driver Research: Learn, Share, and Help End This Deadly Epidemic." 2017: nsc.org/learn/NSC-Initiatives/Pages/distracted-driving-research-studies.aspx.

The University of Utah. "Drivers on Cell Phones Are as Bad as Drunks." 2016: archives.unews.utah.edu/news_releases/drivers-on-cell-phones-are-as-bad-as-drunks/.

D. L. Strayer, et al. "A Comparison of the Cell Phone Driver and the Drunk Driver." *Human Factors*. 2006 Summer; 48(2): 381–91.

Deane Alban. "The Cognitive Costs of Multitasking." Be Brain Fit: bebrainfit.com/cognitive-costs-multitasking/.

Marie Kondo. *The Life-Changing Magic of Tidying Up: The Japanese Art of Decluttering and Organizing.* 2014.

Joseph Pizzorno. *The Toxin Solution: How Hidden Poisons in the Air, Water, Food, and Products We Use Are Destroying Our Health—AND WHAT WE CAN DO TO FIX IT.* 2018.

David Ewing Duncan. "Chemicals Within Us." *National Geographic.* 2006.

Anthony Samsel, Stephanie Seneff. "Glyphosate's Suppression of Cytochrome P450 Enzymes and Amino Acid Biosynthesis by the Gut Microbiome: Pathways to Modern Diseases." *Entropy* 2013, 15(4), 1416–1463; doi.org/10.3390/e15041416.

World Health Organization International Agency for Research on Cancer. *Glyphosate.* March 2015: monographs.iarc.fr/wp-content/upoads/2018/06/mono112-110.pdf.

Mark Hyman, MD. *Food: What the Heck Should I Eat?* 2018. Good section on sugar and sweeteners.

Karyn Shanks, MD. "Simple Is Better: The 'Rule of Threes.'" 2017: karynshanksmd.com/2017/12/04/simple-is-better-rule-of-threes/.

Ben Johnson. *Using the Rule of Three for Learning.* Edutopia: George Lucas Educational Foundation. April 27, 2016: edutopia.org/blog/using-rule-three-learning-ben-johnson.

CHAPTER THREE

The HeartMath Institute: Heartmath.org.

Joseph Chilton Pearce. *The Heart-Mind Matrix: How the Heart Can Teach the Mind New Ways to Think.* 2012.

Sebastian Franke and Hill Kulu. "Cause-specific Mortality by Partnership Status: Simultaneous Analysis Using Longitudinal Data from England and Wales." *J Epi Comm Health, BMJ.* 2018; 72(9): dx.doi.org/10.1136/jech-2017-210339.

Brené Brown. *Daring Greatly; Rising Strong.*

Julianne Holt-Lunstad, et al. "Social Relationships and Mortality Risk: A Meta-analytic Review." *PLoS Med.* 2010 Jul; 7(7): e1000316.

Kory Floyd, et al. "Kissing in Marital and Cohabitating Relationships: Effects on Blood Lipids, Stress, and Relationship Satisfaction." *Western Journal of Communication.* Volume 73, 2009, issue 2.

Light KC, et al. "More Frequent Partner Hugs and Higher Oxytocin Levels Are Linked to Lower Blood Pressure and Heart Rate in Premenopausal Women." *Biol Psychol.* 2005 Apr; 69(1): 5–21: ncbi.nlm.nih.gov/pubmed/15740822.

Catherine Haslam et al. "Social Connectedness and Health." In *Encyclopedia of Geropsychology*, pp. 1–10. 2015: researchgate.net/publication/302472164_Social_Connectedness_and_Health. Review of the literature on Social Connectedness and multiple measures of health.

Katherine Harmon. "Social Ties Boost Survival by 50 Percent: A Meta-Study Covering More Than 300,000 Participants Across All Ages Reveals That Adults Get a 50 Percent Boost in Longevity if They Have a Solid Social Network." *Scientific American.* July 28, 2010: scientificamerican.com/article/relationships-boost-survival/. Nice review of powerful meta-analysis on the health benefits of social connection.

Isobel E. M. Evans, et al. "Social Isolation, Cognitive Reserve, and Cognition in Healthy Older People." *PLos One.* 2018; 13(8): e0201008:ncbi.nlm.nih.gov/pmc/articles/PMC6097646/. Recent review of an older population of 3593 healthy individuals followed for two years, demonstrated a correlation between living a socially active lifestyle and preservation of cognitive function and reserve.

Angela R. Sutin, et al. "Loneliness and Risk of Dementia." 26 October 2018. *J Gerontology: Series B*, gby112: doi.org/10.1093/geronb/gby112.

Tjalling Jan Holwerda, et al. "Feelings of Loneliness, but Not Social Isolation, Predict Dementia Onset: Results from the Amsterdam Study of the Elderly" *AMSTEL*. 2013, Volume 85, issue 2: dx.doi.org/10.1136/jnnp-2012-302755.

Brett Friedler, M.S. et al. "One Is the Deadliest Number: The Detrimental Effects of Social Isolation on Cerebrovascular Diseases and Cognition." *Acta Neuropathol*. 2015 Apr; 129(4): 493–509: ncbi.nlm.nih.gov/pmc/articles/PMC4369164/.

B. Egolf, et al. "The Roseto Effect: A 50-Year Comparison of Mortality Rates." *Am J Public Health*. 1992 August; 82(8): 1089-1092: ncbi.nim.nih.gov/pmc/articles/PMC1695733/.

Nancy J. Donovan, et al. "Association of Higher Cortical Amyloid Burden with Loneliness in Cognitively Normal Older Adults." *JAMA Psychiatry*. 2016 Dec 1; 73(12): 1230-1237: europepmc.org/articles/PMC5257284/.

Grossman and Leroux. "A New Roseto Effect." *Chicago Tribune*. October 11, 1996.

Jerf W. K. Yeung, et al. "Volunteering and Health Benefits in General Adults: Cumulative Effects and Forms." *BMC Public Health*. 2018; 18: 8: ncbi.nlm.nih.gov/pmc/articles/PMC5504679/.

Marianne Williamson. *A Return to Love: Reflections on the Principles of "A Course in Miracles."* 1996.

Leader Dogs for the Blind: leaderdog.org.

Victor J. Strecher. *Life on Purpose: How Living for What Matters Most Changes Everything*. 2016. Great exploration of the connection between purposeful living and the latest scientific evidence on quality of life and longevity.

Viktor Frankl. *Man's Search for Meaning*. 1946.

Desmond Tutu. *The Book of Forgiveness: The Fourfold Path for Healing Ourselves and Our World.* 2015.

Kathleen A. Lawler, et al. "The Unique Effects of Forgiveness on Health: An Exploration of Pathways." *Journal of Behavioral Medicine.* April 2005, Volume 28, Issue 2, pp 157–167: springer.com/article/10.1007/s10865-3665-2.

Laura Redwine, et al. "A Pilot Randomized Study of a Gratitude Journaling Intervention on HRV and Inflammatory Biomarkers in Stage B Heart Failure Patients." *Psychosom Med.* 2016 Jul–Aug; 78(6): 667–676: ncbi.nlm.nih.gov/pmc/articles/PMC4927423/.

Randy A. Sansone, MD and Lori A. Sansone, MD. "Gratitude and Well Being: The Benefits of Appreciation." *Psychiatry.* 2010 Nov; 7(11): 18–22: ncbi.nim.nih.gov/pmc/articles/PMC3010965.

Rod Stryker. *The Four Desires: Creating a Life of Purpose, Happiness, Prosperity, and Freedom.* 2011. Rod's "Healing the Heart" meditation is a beautiful iteration of the many heart-focused meditations I've enjoyed over the years.

CHAPTER FOUR

Jon Kabat-Zinn. *Wherever You Go, There You Are: Mindfulness Meditation in Everyday Life.* 2005. Excellent classic primer on the mindfulness approach to meditation.

Anne Lamott. *Plan B: Further Thoughts on Faith.* 2006.

Joan Borysenko, PhD. Keynote presentation given at the Institute for Functional Medicine Annual International Conference in San Diego. 2016.

Joan Z. Borysenko, PhD. *Fried: Why You Burn Out and How to Revive.* 2011.

Tara Brach. *Radical Acceptance: Awakening the Love That Heals Fear and Shame.* 2003. A Buddhist perspective on cultivating equanimity.

Amy Cuddy. *Presence: Bringing Your Boldest Self to Your Biggest Challenges.* 2015.

Amy Cuddy. "Your Body Language May Shape Who You Are." TED: Ideas Worth
Spreading:
ted.com/talks/amy_cuddy_your_body_language_shapes_who_you_are?language=en.

Kelly McGonigal, PhD. *The Upside of Stress.* 2016.

Suresh I. S. Rattan, Marios Kyriazi, editors. *The Science of Hormesis in Health and Longevity.*
2018. Comprehensive review of mild stress-induced physiological hormesis and its
role in the maintenance and promotion of good health.

Leonard A. Wisneski, *The Scientific Basis of Integrative Medicine,* 2nd edition, 2009.

Hans Selye, MD. "Stress and the General Adaptation Syndrome." *BMJ,* June 17, 1950.

Alia J. Crum, et al. "Improving Stress without Reducing Stress: The Benefits of Stress Is
Enhancing Mindset in Both Challenging and Threatening Contexts." 2014:
mbl.stanford.edu/sites/default/files/crumental_mindsetthreatchallenge_8.27.16.pdf.

Richardson S, et al. "Meta-Analysis of Perceived Stress and Its Association with Incident
Coronary Artery Disease." *Am J Cardiol.* 2012 Dec 15; 110(12): 1711–6:
ncbi.nlm.nih.gov/pubmed/22975465.

Hermann Nabi, et al. "Increased Risk of Coronary Heart Disease Among Individuals
Reporting Adverse Impact of Stress on Their Health: The Whitehall 11 Prospective
Cohort Study." *Eur Heart J* (2013): ncbi.nlm.nih.gov/pubmed/2380458.

Keller A, et al. "Does the Perception That Stress Affects Health Matter? The Association
with Health And Mortality." *Health Psychol.* 2012 Sep; 31 (5): 677–84:
ncbi.nlm.nih.gov/pubmed/22201278.

Kenneth Pelletier, *Mind as Healer, Mind as Slayer,* 1977. Classic text on stress.

Robert Sapolsky, *Why Zebras Don't Get Ulcers,* 2004.

Victoria K. Lee, MD. "Fatal Distraction." *Can Fam Physician.* 2013 Jul; 59(7): 723–725:
ncbi.nlm.nih.gov/pmc/articles/PMC3710028/

Angela Duckworth, Grit: *The Power of Passion and Perseverance,* 2016.

Amy Cuddy, *Presence: Bringing Your Boldest Self to Your Biggest Challenges*, 2015.

Rick Hanson. *Resilient: 12 Tools for Transforming Everyday Experiences into Lasting Happiness.* 2018. Further reading and practical wisdom for creating a strong center.

CHAPTER FIVE

Leonard A. Wisneski, *The Scientific Basis of Integrative Medicine*, 2nd edition, 2009.

Arianna Huffington. *The Sleep Revolution: Transforming Your Life, One Night at a Time.* 2017.

Colten HR, Altevogt, BM, editors. "Sleep Disorders and Sleep Deprivation: An Unmet Public Health Problem." Institute of Medicine (US) Committee on Sleep Medicine and Research; Washington (DC): *National Academies Press* (US), 2006: ncbi.nlm.nih.gov/books/NBK19956/.

Xie L. et al. "Sleep Drives Metabolite Clearance from the Adult Brain." *Science.* 2013 Oct 18; 342(6156): 373–7: ncbi.nlm.nih.gov/pubmed/24136970.

Andrew R. Mendelsohn and James W. Larrick. "Sleep Facilitates Clearance of Metabolites from the Brain: Glymphatic Function in Aging and Neurodegenerative Diseases." *Rejuvenation Research,* Vol. 16, No. 6: liebertpub.com/doi/abs/10.1089/ref.2013.1530.

Till Roenneberg and Martha Merrow. "The Circadian Clock and Human Health." *Current Biology.* Volume 26, Issue 10, 23 May 2016, p R432–43: sciencedirect.com/science/article/pii/S0960982216303335. More science on the connection of the internal circadian clock and health.

Bjorn Rasch and Jan Born. "About Sleep's Role in Memory." *Physiol Rev.* 2013 Apr; 93(2): 681–766: ncbi.nlm.nih.gov/pmc/articles/PMC3768102/.

Kate Porcheret, PhD, et al. "Psychological Effect of an Analogue Traumatic Event Reduced by Sleep Deprivation." *Sleep.* Volume 38, Issue 7, 1 July 2015, pg 1017–1025: doi.org/10.5665/sleep.4802.

Mindy Engle-Friedman. "The Effects of Sleep Loss on Capacity and Effort." *Sleep Science*. Volume 7, Issue 4, December 2014, pages 213–224: sciencedirect.com/science/article/pii/S1984006314000583.

National Sleep Foundation. "Shift Work Disorder." sleepfoundation.org/shift-work/content/living-coping-shift-work-disorder. Review and resources to address problems associated with shift work-related sleep disorder.

Christian Benedict, et al. Gut Microbiota and Glucometabolic Alterations in Response to Recurrent Partial Sleep Deprivation in Normal-Weight Young Individuals." *Molecular Metabolism*. Vol 5, Issue 2, Dec 2016, pg 1175–1186: sciencedirect.com/science/articles/pii/S2212877816301934.

Jason R. Anderson. "A Preliminary Examination of Gut Microbiota, Sleep, and Cognitive Flexibility in Healthy Older Adults." *Sleep Medicine*. Vol 38, Oct 2017, pg 104–107: sciencedirect.com/science/article/pii/S1380045717303179.

Max Hirshkowitz, PhD, et al. "National Sleep Foundation's Sleep Time Duration Recommendations: Methodology and Results Summary." *Sleep Health*, March 2015: Volume 1, Issue 1, Pages 40–43: sleephealthjournal.org/article/S2352-7218%2815%2900015-7/fulltext.

Huber, Reto, et al. Exposure to Pulsed High-Frequency Electromagnetic Field During Waking Affects Human Sleep EEG." *NeuroReport*: October 20, 2000, Volume 11, Issue 15, p 3321–3325: journals.lww.com/neuroreport/Fulltext/2000/10200/Exposure_to_pulsed_high_frequency_electromagnetic.12.aspx.

The National Institute for Play: nifplay.org. Compendium of current research articles on the benefits of play: scholoarpedia.org/article/Encyclopedia: *Play Science*.

Norman Cousins. *Anatomy of an Illness: As Perceived by the Patient*. First edition, 1979. A ground-breaking classic on combating life-threatening illness through humor and patient agency in their own care.

CHAPTER SIX

Katy Bowman. *Move Your DNA*, 2015.

John Durant. *The Paleo Manifesto: Ancient Wisdom for Lifelong Health.* 2014.

Aviroop Biswas, et al. "Sedentary Time and Its Association with Risk for Disease Incidence, Mortality, and Hospitalization in Adults: A Systematic Review and Meta-analysis." *Ann Intern Med.* 2015; 162(2):123-132. doi:10.7326/M14-1651.

"Sedentary Behavior: Emerging Evidence for a New Health Risk." *Mayo Clinic Proceedings.* 2010 Volume 85(12); 1138–1141: mayoclinicproceedings.org/article/S0025-6196(11)60368-6/abstract.

Ashish Sharma, MD. et al. "Exercise for Mental Health." *Prim Care Companion J Clin Psychiatry.* 2006; 8(2): 106: ncbi.nlm.nih.gov/pmc/articles/PMC1470658.

Katy Bowman. *Don't Just Sit There*, 2015.

Amy Cuddy. *Presence: Bringing Your Boldest Self to Your Biggest Challenges.* 2015.

Judith Blackstone, PhD. *Belonging Here: A Guide for the Spiritually Sensitive Person.* 2012.

Stephen Kotler. *The Rise of Superman: Decoding the Science of Ultimate Human Performance.* 2014.

James Gordon, MD. *Unstuck: Your Guide to the Seven-Stage Journey Out of Depression*, 2008.

Rob C. van Lummel, et al. "The Instrumented Sit-to-Stand Test (iSTS) Has Greater Clinical Relevance than the Manually Recorded Sit-to-Stand Test in Older Adults." *PLoS One.* 2016; 11(7): e0157968: ncbi.nlm.nih.gov/pmc/articles/PMC4938439/.

Michael J. Boyle. *New Functional Training for Sports.* 2016.

James Driver. *HIIT—High Intensity Interval Training Explained.* 2012.

Christopher McDougall. *Born to Run: A Hidden Tribe, Superathletes, and the Greatest Race the World Has Never Seen.* 2009.

Matthew W. Sanford. *Waking: A Memoir of Trauma and Transcendence.* 2006. A story of transformational movement following traumatic injury.

CHAPTER SEVEN

Eisenberg, David M, Burgess, Jonathan D. "Nutrition Education in an Era of Global Obesity and Diabetes: Thinking Outside the Box." *Academic Medicine.* 2015: 90(7): 854–860. Doi: 10.1097/ACM.0000000000000682.

William Davis, MD. *Wheat Belly: Lose the Wheat, Lose the Weight, and Find Your Path Back to Health.* 2011.

David Perlmutter, MD. *Grain Brain: The Surprising Truth about Wheat, Carbs, and Sugar—Your Brain's Silent Killers.* Revised edition, 2018.

Mark Hyman, MD. *The Blood Sugar Solution: The UltraHealthy Program for Losing Weight, Preventing Disease, and Feeling Great Now!* 2012.

Loren Cordain. *The Paleo Diet: Lose Weight and Get Healthy by Eating the Food You Were Designed to Eat.* 2001. Classic work on optimal human diets based on anthropological food science.

Karyn Shanks, MD. Protein: a Primer. 2018: karynshanksmd.com/2018/12/10/protein-a-primer/.

Michael Pollan. *Food Rules.* 2009.

Agalaee Jacobs, MS, RD. *Digestive Health with REAL Food: A Practical Guide to an Anti-Inflammatory, Nutrient-Dense Diet for IBS and Other Digestive Issues,* Updated and Expanded. 2018.

National Resources Defense Council. *The Smart Seafood Buying Guide*: nrdc.org/stories/smart-seafood-buying-guide.

Leo Galland. "The Gut Microbiome and the Brain." *J Med Food.* 2014 Dec 1; 17(12): 1261–1272: ncbi.nlm.nih.gov/pmc/articles/PMC4259177/.

Mark Hyman, MD. *Food: What the Heck Should I Eat?* 2018. A nice review of Functional Medicine principles applied to food and nutrition.

Sarah Ballantyne, PhD. *The Paleo Approach: Reverse Autoimmune Disease and Heal Your Body.* 2014.

Sarah Ballantyne, PhD. *The Paleo Approach Cookbook: A Detailed Guide to Heal Your Body and Nourish Your Soul.* 2014.

CHAPTER EIGHT

Norman Doidge, MD. *The Brain's Way of Healing: Remarkable Discoveries and Recoveries from the Frontiers of Neuroplasticity.* 2015.

Norman Doidge, MD. *The Brain That Changes Itself: Stories of Personal Triumph from the Frontiers of Brain Science.* 2007.

Robert Kegan and Lisa Laskow Lahey. *How the Way We Talk Can Change the Way We Work: Seven Languages for Transformation.* 2000.

Don Miguel Ruiz. *The Four Agreements: A Practical Guide to Personal Freedom, A Toltec Wisdom Book.* 2001. Explores how making assumptions keeps us stuck and unhappy.

CHAPTER NINE

Joshua D. Rosenblat, et al. "Inflamed Moods: A Review of the Interactions between Inflammation and Mood Disorders." *Progress in Neuro-Psychopharmacology and Biological Psychiatry.* Volume 53, 4 August 2014, pages 23–34: sciencedirect.com/science/article/pii/S0278584614000141.

David R. Hawkins, MD, PhD. *Power vs Force (Author's Official Revised Addition): The Hidden Determinants of Human Behavior.* 2012.

Candice Pert. *Molecules of Emotion: Why You Feel the Way You Feel.* 1997. Classic text on the biology of emotions.

Judith Orloff, MD. *The Empath's Survival Guide: Life Strategies for Sensitive People.* 2017.

Susan Cain. *Quiet: The Power of Introverts in a World That Can't Stop Talking.* 2012.

Abraham H. Maslow. *A Theory of Human Motivation.* 1943.

Rippentrop, Betsy. *The Complete Idiot's Guide to the Chakras: Renew Your Life Force with the Chakras Seven Energy Centers.* 2009. Concise exploration of the Vedic chakra model of emotional anatomy.

Carolyn Myss. *The Anatomy of the Spirit: The Seven Stages of Power and Healing.* 1997. A classic exploration of the use of emotional anatomy to heal.

Sonia Choquette. *The Psychic Pathway: A Workbook for Reawakening the Voice of Your Soul.* 1995. Classic exploration of how emotions bring forth intuitive wisdom.

Bessel van der Kolk, MD. *The Body Keeps the Score: Brain, Mind, and Body in the Healing of Trauma.* 2014.

James S. Gordon, MD. *The Transformation: Discovering Wholeness and Healing After Trauma.* 2019.

CHAPTER TEN

Huston Smith. *Tales of Wonder: Adventures Chasing the Divine, an Autobiography.* 2009. My mentor.

Abraham H. Maslow. *Religions, Values, and Peak-Experiences.* 1994.

Albert Einstein. *Living Philosophies.* 1931.

Jake Abrahamson. "The Science of Awe." *Sierra.* Nov/Dec, 2014: sierraclub.org/sierra/2014-6-november-december/feature/science-awe.

Stellar, Jennifer E. et al. "Positive Affect and Markers of Inflammation: Discrete Positive Emotions Predict Lower Levels of Inflammatory Cytokines." *Emotion.* Vol 15(2): Apr. 2015: ncbi.nlm.nih.gov/pubmed/25603133.

CHAPTER ELEVEN

Sydney Baker MD. *Detoxification and Healing: The Key to Optimal Health.* 2003. Creator of the famous "Three Tack Rule."

Theodore Roosevelt. "Citizenship in a Republic." Speech at the Sorbonne; April 23, 1910: Theodore-roosevelt.com/images/research/speeches/maninthearena.pdf.

INDEX

ABOUT THE AUTHOR

Dr. Karyn Shanks is a physician, teacher, and author of *Heal: A Nine-Stage Roadmap to Recover Energy, Reverse Chronic Illness, and Claim the Potential of a Vibrant New You.*

Karyn believes that health and vitality are essential for the highest expression of our human potential and that the bones of healing are in what we do for ourselves. During twenty-eight-years of medical practice she has helped thousands of clients with chronic illness to heal, and to regain their hope, their energy, and their life's potential. Listening passionately to their stories while fully engaged with her own life-school of learning, Dr. Shanks has developed *The Nine Domains of Healing* roadmap that synthesizes what she has learned to be true: that healing is always possible, that it is within everyone's grasp, and that it ultimately comes from within. Whether working with clients suffering from debilitating disease, or those who feel there is more and want to feel like themselves again, she shares her extensive knowledge and experiences in a way that is approachable and leads clients into change that is doable. Guiding, teaching, and cheering on her clients (also kicking them in the butt when necessary!), Karyn is a mentor who connects with people and reminds them of what is possible.

Dr. Shanks received her medical degree from the University of Chicago and completed her training in Internal Medicine at the University of Iowa. Board certified in Internal Medicine and Functional Medicine, she is also a founding diplomat of the American Board of Integrative and Holistic Medicine. She will say, though, that her greatest teacher has been Life School, the profound lessons she has learned as a person, a physician, and a patient herself. She has integrated those lessons with the science, cultural wisdom, and experiential knowledge gleaned from her extensive work. She is the founder and director of The Center for Medicine and Healing Arts in Iowa City. She is sought out nationally as a healer by her clients and as a mentor by Functional Medicine practitioners. In addition to numerous articles in the Huffington Post, Holstee, Thrive Global, and others, as well as her own weekly blog and email series "Dear Ones," she is also the author of *Big Energy: How We Reclaim Our Health, Our Vitality Our Lives, Let Go: The Nine Domains of Healing, Part One,* and *Love: The Nine Domains of Healing, Part Two.*

Karyn lives in Iowa City with her husband and dogs. She is most proud of her two sons, beautifully launched and landed in their own lives. She loves her many playgrounds—the woods, gym, yoga studio, her back deck, and her writing room.

Visit Karyn's work at www.KarynShanksMD.com.

Contact her at Karyn@KarynShanksMD.com.

Sign up for her weekly *Dear Ones* emails at www.KarynShanksMD.com/sign-up/.

Join Karyn and like-minded seekers of vibrant health in her exclusive Facebook group, *Grit and Grace*: www.facebook.com/groups/gritandgracecommunity. This is where we share the hard work of self-care: our struggles, insights, and our stories.

Made in the USA
Monee, IL
29 June 2023

38057556R00201